AN INTERMITTENT FASTING GUIDE FOR WOMEN OVER 50

BOOST BRAIN HEALTH, LOSE WEIGHT, IMPROVE METABOLISM, AND REGAIN VITALITY WHILE STILL EATING THE FOODS YOU LOVE

LESLEY LEACH BSN, RN CPT

CONTENTS

Just For You

A FREE GIFT TO MY READERS.
TOP 12 FAT LOSS FOODS WITH RECIPES!!

Just Scan the QR Code and download the PDF.

INTRODUCTION

> *Fasting is the single greatest natural healing therapy. It is nature's ancient, universal 'remedy' for many problems.*
>
> — ELSON HAAS, M.D.

Did you know that 38 percent of American women resort to hormone replacement therapy to deal with their menopausal aftereffects (Fletcher & Colditz, 2002)? Even when this replacement therapy has been shown to increase the risk of several types of cancers and cardiovascular disorders, women turn to it to deal with their hormonal dilemmas (Rymer et al., 2003). Another even larger group of women turn to fad diets to deal with weight gain and other menopause-related issues. These restrictive diets may cut down a few pounds off the scale, but these results are temporary, and the side effects that come along with it make this process a lot less fun. Additionally, the food restrictions mandated by these diet plans can end up causing more harm to your physical and cognitive health than good. What if I told you there is a way that allows weight loss, improves mental health, boosts organ function, and improves metabolism, all without implementing strict diet restrictions? That method is intermittent fasting (IF). IF offers all of these benefits without having you compromise on your diet and routine.

IF is the eating pattern that involves eating meals only at a specific time each day. This allows you to manage your weight, maintain energy levels, sustain bone health, and evade the risk of chronic health disorders. Skipping entire meals means your daily calorie intake is lowered so much that you don't need to worry about calories during meal times. The risk of losing muscle mass that is high in dieting plans is sufficiently lowered in the case of IF. The feelings of hunger and starvation common in restrictive dieting are also managed in IF. This means that there is no chance that your hunger hormones will be affected as they do in dieting. Lastly, intermittent fasting is known to reduce belly fat, which makes it an excellent option for women who have been struggling with weight management for several years.

Before we get into its details, let's see how the 50s can be a turbulent time for women. The changes accompanied by menopause create fluctuations in hormonal levels. These hormones that keep our organs healthy and our bodies active start lowering as we age. Resultantly, our organ systems start functioning less ideally; there is either a high of something or a low of another. Heart and brain take the greatest hit. A slight loss of efficiency in one organ has a ripple effect on other organs, and this results in a plethora of diseases and disorders.

The blood vessels lose their inherent elasticity with age, and the pressure inside them gradually mounts. Stress and weight are two contributing factors here, which are also high at this age. All of these lead to blood pressure issues and a major risk of cardiovascular diseases. The fact that this condition progresses in a stealth mode makes it even more dangerous. Perhaps this is the reason why Ischaemic heart diseases are the leading cause of death in the world, accounting for 16% of the deaths (as of 2019) (McCarthy, 2020).

Accumulation of cholesterol in the blood vessels is also a contributing factor to these heart-related disorders. Cholesterol buildup is a slow process, and it becomes apparent in the late 50s. Besides blood pressure and cholesterol, blood sugar levels also start to get unmanageable in the 50s. There are multiple risk factors for diabetes, including lifestyle, eating habits, and family history, but around age 50 and above, our bodies no longer have the stamina to bear such sugar levels, and this can result in diabetes and a group of related health problems.

Fifty years of work and physical activity take a toll on our skeletal system as well. This results in the wearing and tearing of the cartilage between bones, thus making our movements more restricted and painful. A drop in the production of estrogen hormone in women affects bone density. This means that the bones get brittle, and there is a higher risk of osteoporosis development. With advancing age, the risk of cancer development becomes even more significant. Women over 50 especially need to screen for breast cancer and colon cancer. Women at this age are also susceptible to infections because of the waning immune system. Lastly, hormonal imbalance is the biggest issue in this age group. This stress will, in turn, affect their physical health even more, and this can initiate a never-ending cycle of unhealthiness in the body and mind.

A closer look at all of these age-related problems highlights a vital issue, i.e., poor weight management, and its role in exacerbating these health issues. When women start experiencing age-related problems like low energy levels, muscle stiffness, and bone weakness, they resort to high-caloric foods thinking that they will help them cover their health crisis. However, this high-calorie diet results in them gaining extra weight that acts as a catalyst for the development of several metabolic disorders (heart disease, stroke, and type 2 diabetes). Simply resorting to a high-calorie diet is not the solution. What these women require is a diet plan that allows them to consume nutrient-rich foods that are sufficient to meet their energy requirements and to keep their weight in check.

By "diet plan," I don't mean the exclusion of specific foods from the diet. I mean a diet that allows you to eat everything you like but in a way that helps keep your weight in check, and this is where Intermittent Fasting (IF) comes in.

Intermittent fasting is the ultimate solution for you if you:

- are struggling with weight management.
- are dealing with post-menopausal hormonal imbalance and the accompanying physiological changes.
- have continuous brain fog.
- want to manage your blood sugar levels, blood cholesterol levels, and blood pressure.
- want to see yourself as a strong, self-confident woman with a positive body image.

This book will help you discover the miracles of IF and how it can help you regain your strength and health. I will walk you through the methods of IF and provide you with customized meal plans. You will discover the dos and don'ts of IF that could help you achieve better results. Besides this, we will also focus on the importance of working out during fasting and how it could amplify the benefits of IF for you.

You see, most of the literature out there focuses on a single IF technique, which makes it difficult for readers to compare and choose a single technique that suits them. Also, most of these books are a compilation of ideal case scenarios and expert opinions on IF but lack the inclusion of personal experiences. I, however, have personal experience with IF, and I have had my fair share of successes and failures with my weight management journey. In my 18 years as a nurse and 19 years as a fitness professional, I have gained a close insight into what women in their 50s go through regarding their physical and mental health and how unhealthy lifestyle choices weigh heavily on their health, and I want to help them achieve optimal health regardless of their age.

Remember, age is just a number, and you should never allow it to claim your confidence, health, and energy. Through a carefully selected combination of nutrition and exercise, you can regain your health and reclaim your frisky 50s.

1

WHAT IS INTERMITTENT FASTING: THE SCIENCE MADE EASY

During the mid-19th century, dieting was thought to be the ultimate solution for everyone looking to manage their weight or restrict calories. Everyone from fashion-conscious teenagers to older adults who wanted to defeat their obesity turned to restrictive dieting plans, but dieting has its disadvantages that not everyone can handle. These disadvantages have slowly shifted people's attention to IF. IF has gradually gained popularity over the last few years, and its multiple advantages, simplicity, and flexibility have led it to overtake strict dieting as the primary eating style for men and women all over the world. So, before we delve deeper, let's first understand what IF is, how it works, and how it is different from other eating patterns.

WHAT IS INTERMITTENT FASTING?

As the name suggests, IF is the eating plan that cycles between normal eating and fasting. "Normal eating" here does not mean eating voraciously. Unlike dieting plans, IF focuses on when to eat rather than what to eat. The idea is to promote healthy eating habits and to give the body a break from continuous food digestion. This break allows several vital organs, including the brain, intestines, liver, and pancreas, to take the much-needed rest. Fasting most of the day and then eating only for a specific part of the day allows you to burn fat and reverse damage caused by mindless eating. Besides, IF has also been known for its potential to lower the risk of certain age-related diseases and disorders.

The idea behind IF is to prolong the break between meals so that your body gets sufficient time to burn all of those previously ingested calories and start burning fats before the next batch of calories comes in. Unlike strict dieting, IF is a relatively more straightforward meal plan with a variety of techniques to choose from and no special meal planning and preparations involved. This is what makes it the most popular fitness trend around the world. IF promotes healthy eating, providing nutrition and acting as a remedy for most of your health issues.

HISTORY OF INTERMITTENT FASTING

You might think that IF is a new method, but that's not true. IF has gained popularity recently as a lifestyle and fitness trend, but the concept is not new. In prehistoric times, hunter-gatherer societies fasted because they had no other choice. It took time to hunt animals, and even when animals were available, they were never enough to feed the whole tribe. When they started gathering and storing fruits and berries, they had a good supply of food in the summers, but they still had to fast in the winters. This suggests that humans have innate capabilities to tolerate hunger for several hours and days. It was only after the man learned to farm that he started eating several meals a day. But still, it was easier to maintain a healthy weight since life was hard and luxuries were scarce.

Besides food scarcity, several other reasons make people fast. People fast for religious reasons, too, since they are taught that fasting is a way to cleanse souls and keep evil at bay. Ancient Greeks thought that having a full stomach acted as a cue for demonic entities, while Muslims are of the view that overeating makes them lethargic and less keen to worship God. Fasting is an important part of the Muslim faith, and they fast from dawn to dusk every day for a whole month (Ramadan). I lived in Dubai at the time; thank you, Chris Walker, and I was blessed to observe this practice firsthand. It was a wondrous experience and will stay with me always.

This was the very first time that I got to see the benefits that fasting can have on people's health and mood.

The same teachings were propagated by Christianity and Buddhism. The old testaments of these religions indicate that. With time, churches started customary observance of fasting practices partially to promote the spirit of penance and self-cleansing of the soul. Ancient Greek thinkers like Hippocrates and Plato supported and practiced fasting too. They were of the view that fasting is an easy way to cure several types of illnesses and to increase mental abilities.

Fasting started to gain importance in the scientific world in the late 1880s when several people started to share their experiences with fasting. By the 1950s, several types of research were being conducted to decipher the medical effects of fasting. The first research of this kind was conducted by Ancel Keys and his co-worker at the University of Minnesota. They collected data from 32 volunteers who practiced intermittent fasting for eight months (Tobey, 1951). Before that, research was conducted in the 1940s to gauge the effects of calorie restriction on mice. The study showed a relative increase in the life span of mice due to fasting. Similar research showed the same results for other animals like fish and dogs, yet data regarding its effects on human life span was limited.

Fasting for the sake of weight management was introduced by Folin and Denis in 1914.

In the 2000s, Bert Herring and his wife proposed a fast-five approach to IF. This was based on a 19/5 pattern which allowed a five-hour eating window. This rather flexible fasting plan gained much popularity. Since then, several types and variations of intermittent fasting have been introduced, all of which provide more or less similar results. The first style of IF was proposed by a fitness coach, Michael O'Donnell, in 2007. He named it the Two Meal System, a meal plan that includes eating two meals per day. In the same year, an IF program was popularized by Martin Berkhan by the name of Leangains. He came up with the idea of the 16/8 pattern, which is a popular regimen to date. Lastly, a Canadian nutritionist, Brad Pilon, proposed a version of IF named Eat-Stop-Eat. This regimen consists of one or two full-day fasts per week. This also includes exercising at the beginning of the 24-hour fast to maximize the benefits of fasting.

In addition to these versions of IF, several other versions have been introduced over time, the details of which I'll discuss later, along with their precautions and meal plans.

THE SCIENCE OF INTERMITTENT FASTING

Research is still underway to decipher and explain the miraculous effects of IF on the modern world. However, sufficient research reveals that IF has a significant impact on weight management, building muscles, and reducing the risk of diabetes. Let's see how.

Weight Loss

Weight loss is one of the goals of IF, and this is brought on by several factors. Firstly, restricting eating to a specific time window(s) per day naturally decreases daily calorie intake. Additionally, the decreased levels of insulin in the blood influence metabolism to kick-start the consumption of stored fats for energy production. The removal of this accumulated fat contributes to weight loss.

How Do We Gain This Weight?

When you eat food, the carbohydrate component in it gets broken down into tiny glucose molecules. These molecules then enter the blood and get transported to every cell in your body that needs energy. Extra glucose that is not required at the time is stored in the liver (as glycogen) and as fats in the fat cells.

In the case of overeating or eating more than the body's requirement, continuous accumulation and storage of glycogen and fats result in you gaining weight. A sedentary lifestyle aggravates this weight gain even more.

How Fasting Comes to the Rescue?

It usually takes 10 to 12 hours for an inactive person to exhaust all of the energy derived from the previous meal. But an average person doesn't wait this long to eat the next meal.

So, before the last energy is used up, another batch of glucose comes in and creates an energy surplus, which ultimately leads to weight gain.

The idea of IF is to tackle this very issue. Not only IF prolongs the gap between the two successive meals, but it also creates a calorie deficit. When that happens, the body starts consuming the stored fats to derive energy. This fat is moved out of the fat cell, converted by complex processes into glucose, and then used up in running normal body functions, including digestion, breathing, movement, and brain responsiveness. This process, when employed, periodically contributes to weight loss.

Muscle Building

Have you ever heard of Human Growth Hormone (HGH)? Well, even if you haven't, the name explains it. HGH is the natural hormone that is responsible for promoting growth. It is involved in promoting height, building muscles, and strengthening bones. This hormone is primarily released in childhood, and its production peaks at puberty, but after that, its production is successively decreased. However, research has revealed that fasting stimulates HGH production so much that its production is 1250% increased just after a week of fasting (Kerndt et al., 1982). These elevated levels of HGH are known to promote muscle building, cell repair, and weight loss.

Reduced Diabetes Risk

Every time we eat something, our bodies start working to digest and transform it into useful nutrients. For converting the carbohydrates part of food, a hormone called insulin is produced. This hormone shuttles extra sugar to liver storage. Eating all the time or most of the time during waking hours means that carbs are always high, and so is insulin.

Constant high levels of insulin in the body could lead cells to get desensitized to insulin, and this is where the problem arises. When the body becomes unresponsive to insulin, sugar remains high in the blood, and this can push you to the brink of type 2 diabetes.

IF is an effective way to ensure that the body gets periodic lows and highs of insulin to sustain its insulin sensitivity.

Elevated Brain Performance

IF acts as an exercise for the brain by stimulating the production of the brain's growth stimulators (neurotrophic factors). These growth factors promote the growth and repair of brain cells. Fasting is also known to improve alertness levels and decrease the risk of age-related brain disorders (Gudden et al., 2021).

The latest research in the area of gut health has found a deep connection between the brain and gut health. This has resulted in the concept of the Gut-Brain Axis, which states that gut bacteria have a profound effect on the release of happy hormones (Serotonin, Dopamine, and Endorphins) and also on the development and prevention of neurological disorders. IF deeply affects this Gut-Brain Axis and contributes to clear thinking, elevated mood, and a decreased risk of neurodegenerative disorders. The work by Mattson et al. (2018) talks about the concept of "intermittent metabolic switching," which is the process initiated by periodic intervals of ketosis (fasting and exercising) and recovery (eating and sleeping). This metabolic switching optimizes the brain, promotes longevity, lowers stress, and creates neuroplasticity (the brain's ability to form new neural connections). All of these effects are highly important for people beyond the age of 40 because that's when brain functioning becomes less optimal.

EFFECTIVENESS OF INTERMITTENT FASTING

The effectiveness of fasting has been proved through several year-long studies both in animals and humans. Although this evidence is not as strong in the case of humans as it is in the case of animals, the research proves its efficacy in boosting immune response, lowering bad cholesterol, controlling blood pressure and blood glucose, promoting brain health, and stimulating cellular repair. Despite these potential benefits of intermittent fasting, there is one thing that can sabotage all effort put into IF, i.e., lack of proper knowledge. This can lead some people to overeat during the eating window, eat unhealthy foods or eat too little. IF demands strict adherence to the schedule to tap its maximum benefits. Research has revealed that people who eat at specific times during the day find it easy to follow the IF. Voracious eaters find it hard to adhere to meal schedules (Harvie & Howell, 2017). Seimon et al (2015) reviewed previous research data to conclude that IF has the potential to cause a weight loss of 7-11 pounds over a period of 10 weeks. This review also concluded that IF did not have any effect on the appetite of the fasting group.

When compared with calorie restriction(CR) diets (that limit daily calorie consumption), IF has shown no significant difference in the amount of weight loss. Both IF and CR were found to offer the same results (Rynders et al., 2019).

What Happens to You When You Fast?

We have looked at the potential benefits of IF, but what is it that happens to the human body during fasting? Have you ever wondered how your muscles, brain, and other vital organs react during fasting? What impacts does it have on hormonal balance? Or how do the body's organs work on limited energy reserves?

After 8 Hours of Fasting

After a meal, energy levels are quite high, and every organ gets its full share from the energy reserve, but after about 6 hours, blood glucose levels fall, and the brain gets to decide which organs need to be slowed down to make the glucose reserve last longer. Along with that, the liver starts to send the stored glucose (glycogen) into the blood to meet the energy demand. But even then, after 8 hours, all of the liver reserves are depleted, and the body officially enters the fasting mode. At this point, extra fats are used to generate the much-needed glucose.

Some of these fats are converted into a special type of fuel (called ketone bodies) for the skeletal muscles, heart, and brain cells. Ketone bodies are a better energy source than glucose energy-wise, and IF is an excellent way to increase the production of those ketone bodies.

Technically, each one of us has fasted for eight hours because we usually sleep for eight hours or more. And despite all the above-listed changes that may occur during these eight hours, we don't start to feel hungry after this time. You may have noticed that you are not hungry when you wake up but eat breakfast despite that. We eat because we are taught that eight hours is the maximum time that one should go without food, and so we eat after every eight hours and sometimes in between as well.

After 12 Hours of Fasting

The consumption of stored glucose and fats continues into 12 hours of fasting. However, since the glucagon reserves (in the liver) start to decline, the body begins to transition its demand toward stored fats. The speed of this transition depends on the kind of food that you eat. If this food has more percentage of carbs, the change from glucagon to fats is going to be a slow one. If you eat fat-based foods, the transition from glucagon to fats is a quick one.

After around 12 hours of fasting, the production of growth hormone (HGH) kicks in. As we discussed previously, this hormone boosts fat burning, the repair of cells, and the production of protein in the body. In fact, this hormone is also called the "Anti-aging hormone." So basically, it is one of the main goals of fasting. Around this time, most of the people who are new to IF start feeling hungry.

After 18 Hours of Fasting

By 18 hours, the body is completely running on fats, and the production of fat-based fuel (mostly ketone bodies) is high. A little warm-up exercise can boost their production even more. We have talked about how ketones are a better fuel than carbs, but they have other benefits as well. These ketone bodies are known to increase brain activity, thus contributing to improved levels of alertness and better memory. Also, these molecules act as stress-busters. They do so by accelerating the stress-relieving pathways in the body. This reduces inflammation and repairs the damaged cells in the body.

By this time, the body's reserves of stored glucose (glycogen) start decreasing, and another process starts that biologists call gluconeogenesis. It is the formation of glucose from scratch, which mainly uses waste proteins and fats as the raw material. At this point, HGH makes sure that the system steers clear of muscle proteins. This makes sure that you don't lose muscles to IF.

Another process that starts here is the recycling of the waste in the body. We call it Autophagy (self-eating). I know it sounds intense, but the process is good for the body. The raw materials used here are the dead cells, viruses, and bacteria in your body. Useless proteins that are dumped in the brain and other vital organs get used here. Basically, it's a self-cleansing procedure that lowers the risk of several age-related disorders, especially the ones that affect the brain, like Alzheimer's disease and Parkinson's disease. Clearing the nervous system of useless cells is also helpful in decreasing brain fog. Autophagy slows down the degeneration of heart tissue and the development of several types of cancers.

After 24 Hours of Fasting

After about 24 hours of fasting, the speed of autophagy is exceptionally high, and the process of cellular rejuvenation is occurring at a high pace. It is the lack of this process in adults that triggers neurodegenerative disorders in the brain. Neurodegenerative disorders like Alzheimer's disease and Parkinson's disease are disorders that are characterized by successive loss of brain cells, so IF proves advantageous here by decreasing the risk of such conditions.

While good things may be occurring for you in the body, the glycogen levels are extremely low, and so are your energy levels. At this point, extreme feelings of hunger kick in, but that's just a cue for you to eat. This doesn't mean that you are in danger of any sort. You can skip meals for several hours after that.

After 48 Hours of Fasting

Fasting constantly for 48 hours might seem like an impossible task, but the health benefits at this point are astounding. The HGH levels at this stage are about five times high, and so are the related benefits of fasting. While ketone bodies keep promoting HGH production, there is another important hormone that kicks in, and that's the hunger hormone, ghrelin. Not only ghrelin promotes HGH production, but it also helps in preserving muscle mass and preventing age-related fat accumulation. Also, this hormone promotes the body's natural wound-healing properties and maintains heart health. It is funny how ghrelin affects our psychology to think that we might die of starvation when it's stirring miracles for our health. Hunger at this stage may exist, but it is quite less. Simply drinking a glass of water with some added electrolytes lessens it for hours.

After 72 Hours of fasting

At this point, the insulin (that is released to shuttle extra sugar to the storage section) is at its lowest level since there is no additional sugar in the shuttle. But this also means that insulin sensitivity is at its highest. Remember, keeping the organs sensitive to insulin levels is vital to prevent the development of diabetes.

Besides preventing diabetes, there is a range of health benefits of lowered insulin levels. First, autophagy gets a boost. Second, inflammation is reduced, making you more sensitive to insulin itself. Lastly, the risk of age-related diseases like stroke and cancer is lowered. At the end of a 72-hour fast, the immune system gets rejuvenated since the old immune cells are replaced with new ones.

Such a long fasting duration shuts down all of the body systems that have allowed weakened cells to survive somehow. Resultantly, these cells get shuttled in autophagy, which opens up the chance to form new cells, especially blood cells.

WHO SHOULDN'T TRY INTERMITTENT FASTING?

Considering the unlimited benefits of IF, a vast number of people are using it to attain the required results, but there are also rising concerns among the scientific community that it is only for some. IF has some downsides that not everyone can handle. Let's look at a list of such conditions that can make IF unsuitable for you.

IF is not recommended for:

- Teenagers (below 18 years of age).
- Pregnant women.

- Breastfeeding mothers.
- People who suffer from or are at risk of developing food-related disorders (e,.g. Bulimia Nervosa).
- Voracious eaters (abrupt switching to a fasting lifestyle can hurt mood and energy levels).
- People who have psychological disorders.
- People suffering from sleep issues (trying to sleep on an empty stomach causes brain alertness and keeps us from falling asleep).
- Individuals suffering from stomach issues (constipation, bloating, indigestion).
- Someone on medication that needs to be taken before or after meals.
- Someone with a compromised immune system.

SIDE EFFECTS YOU MIGHT EXPECT FOLLOWING A FASTING LIFESTYLE

With a ton of benefits of IF, there are some side effects as well. And usually, these side effects are common only during the initial fasting days. When done correctly, these side effects can be avoided.

But what exactly are these side effects?

Well, the most common issue is hunger and not just the average amount. IF can lead to increased production of a hormone called cortisol, which can cause one to feel extreme hunger. People who are previously addicted to food may face this side effect more severely. But again, hunger is just a psychological feeling that can be endured.

Another issue that arises with IF is dehydration because most people drink water only during meals. When meals are skipped, so is the water intake. But this problem can be easily avoided by drinking lots of water. You can set reminders for this purpose, or you could have a calorie-free beverage every time you get a hunger pang.

A common problem faced during eating windows is overeating. Voracious eaters often end up eating so much during non-fasting days that it exceeds the calorie loss achieved during the previous fasting session. Some people do stress eating–the stress that has developed due to a lack of calories in the body. To avoid this issue, stress-relieving activities like yoga can help. Eating nutritious yet low-calorie food during the eating window may also prove helpful.

Feeling tired is normal during IF. People new to fasting may face this situation more often because their bodies are not accustomed to fasting. Yoga, meditation, and workouts can help in boosting energy levels.

Celebrity Success Stories

IF has played an essential role in shaping the lives of several people over the years. It has helped them attain a positive self-image and to love themselves all over again. The success story of Gisele Caroline Bündchen is a true testament to IF's efficacy. Bündchen is a Brazilian fashion model, author, and philanthropist. In her book *Lessons, she* has revealed that she uses the 5:2 version of IF. This IF method fits her schedule perfectly as she can eat normally during the first five days of the week, and on the remaining two days, she restricts her calorie intake to a minimum of 500-600 calories. She fasts till lunchtime. This easy-to-follow fasting schedule provides her organs the much-needed rest.

The Lesley Leach Program

Before you start IF, you need to decide a few things. First, you need to find an apparent reason(s) that's making you turn to IF. Having a legit reason will serve as a motivation for you and help determine the subsequent step in your IF journey.

Next, you need to set some realistic goals that you wish to achieve through IF.

Are you fasting to

- lose weight?
- clear brain fog?
- lower diabetes risk?
- decrease inflammation?

Once you have decided that, you need to figure out the kind of IF technique that you should be using.

Lastly, it would be best if you devised a plan for dealing with the side effects of IF. Figure out the most probable side effects that you might face and determine how you will deal with them.

Below is a worksheet of a few important questions that you should know the answer to before starting IF.

What are your reasons for opting for IF?

✎...

✎...

✎...

✎...

Do you feel like these are the valid reason(s)?

✎...

✎...

How long do you want your fasts to be?

✎...

What fluid/electrolytes would you take during the fasting window?

✎...

✎...

✎...

Which exercises would you do during your fasts?

✎...

✎...

✎...

How long do you want your eating windows to be?

✎...

Write a rough meal plan that you would follow during eating windows.

✎...

✎...

✎...

What are the side effects that you would face?

✎...

✎...

How do you plan on dealing with those possible side effects?

✎...

✎...

✎...

✎...

2

INTERMITTENT FASTING EATING SCHEDULES AND BENEFITS

The benefits of IF are numerous, but these can only be gained when you choose the IF plan that is best suited to your body. Additionally, the selection of foods to eat during the eating window should be made with utmost care.

The reason that has made IF so popular among the masses is the fact that it has no restrictions regarding food choices; it is the timing that matters. But the experts are of the view that minimizing the common side effects of IF requires a conscious selection of food. For instance, some people start feeling hungry a few hours into the fasting window. That's because either they eat less or the meals are less fulfilling. To avoid these issues, nutritionists recommend consuming fulfilling meals with low calories but rich in essential nutrients.

FOODS TO EAT

The idea of IF seems so appealing to many because they think that as long as they refrain from eating for a few hours, they are good to eat anything they want during the eating window. Even when this notion is correct, downing a bag of french fries with a cola drink and a tub of ice cream will throw off the theme of IF. Let's look at the list of recommended foods that you should prefer eating during the eating window of your IF.

Lean Proteins

Do you know that proteins take about one to two days to digest completely? This is why taking lean proteins during the eating window is recommended. I don't recommend loading your plates with high-protein foods, but small amounts of lean proteins can make your fasting hours easy to endure. The presence of these proteins will make sure that your body has the ability to sustain and build muscles. Some excellent sources of proteins are:

- chicken
- fish and shellfish
- beans
- legumes
- greek yogurt
- tofu

Beans and legumes not only contain proteins but carbs as well, so they can help sustain your energy levels during fasting hours. Chickpeas and lentils are also known to help lose extra fat. They can serve as an excellent replacement for animal proteins that have unhealthy fats attached to them, even in the case of lean meat. The carbs in lentils cause gradual changes in blood sugar levels, thus creating satiety.

Fruits

Fasting or not-fasting, fruits are always the number one choice of nutritionists when it comes to meal planning. That is because they are loaded with all the goodies; vitamins, minerals, low-carbs, fibers, and good fats.

Vitamins and minerals can help maintain a balanced metabolism during the fast, while the fiber part is a must to maintain bowel health. Fruits that are low in carbs and fats can help attain good levels of blood sugar and blood cholesterol. Fruits are a good source of antioxidants that can help lower the risk of several types of cancer.

Some of the great fruits choices that you could consume during IF are:

- berries (blueberries, cherries, strawberries, and raspberries)
- apples
- plums

- apricots
- pears
- peaches
- oranges

Vegetables

The importance of veggies as an IF food can never be overemphasized. We all hated it when our parents told us to "eat our veggies," but as adults, I think we have made peace with the fact that we have to eat our veggies no matter what. The benefits provided by vegetables are numerous.

Vegetables are known to lower the risk of chronic diseases and help maintain brain health. Broccoli, cauliflower, and brussels sprouts have antioxidant properties which help reduce the cancer risk. The fiber part in them is vital to keep your bowel movements smooth.

Some great vegetable choices include:

- broccoli
- cabbage
- tomatoes
- carrots
- green beans
- kale
- spinach
- carrots

- potatoes

Okay, I know! You might be wondering why I included potatoes in the list when they are famous for causing weight gain. But that's not entirely true. It's not the potatoes that cause weight gain, but the way you consume them. Nutritionists suggest that consuming potatoes in moderation (in the form of healthy dishes, not french fries) can act as a good filling food and help you stay satiated for hours during a fast.

Water

Water doesn't count as food technically, but we cannot move forward before discussing its vitality. You can go for several days without food, but you cannot survive without water as the organs will start to shut down after 3-5 days, give or take, depending on your current state of health. Our bodies can manage to stay on limited glucose reserves or even generate it on their own, but water needs to be replenished constantly. Each of your body organs has different fluid requirements but as a general estimate of how much water your body needs, you can notice the color of your urine. It should always be a light-yellow color. Any fluctuation in its color indicates dehydration, infection, or a disease. Water requirements also differ based on sex, weight, height, lifestyle, and climate. Recommended water requirement for women is 2.7 liters (11-12 cups). You can drink water every 2 hours to meet this demand. Drinking plain water is recommended, but if you find it hard, you can add electrolytes to it or a few slices of lemon and cucumber to it.

Bone Broth

Bone broths are rich in vitamins and minerals. They are also full of collagen, a nutrient that strengthens bones and muscles, rejuvenates skin, and promotes gut health.

Low-Calorie Drinks Such as Unsweetened Coffee

Besides water, there are a few other things that you can have to meet your fluid demand. Since taking anything that has calories in it breaks the fast, technically, you should not have soft drinks, energy drinks, smoothies, or fruit juices. That only leaves you with two options: black, unsweetened coffee or tea (also unsweetened). Coffee is, in fact, great for a fasting body. Not only does it boost the metabolism, but it also increases alertness levels. Also, a cup of black coffee just has like five calories, so there is no chance that it will affect blood sugar levels. Research has also revealed that coffee lowers the risk of cardiac disorders, diabetes, and cancer. It can also help reduce the risk of neurodegenerative disorders like Alzheimer's disease, Parkinson's disease, dementia, and depression (Zhao et al., 2022).

Now there are different schools of thought about having anything with calories in it while fasting. I'm with the mindset that if you can't drink coffee or tea without a little cream, then go for it. Some say you can have up to 30 calories and still reap the benefits of fasting. I personally still have a tablespoon of cream and use a frother to make it nice and whipped. This allows me to get through a 16-20 hour fast with ease. You should also be mindful of artificial sweeteners because despite being a different kind of sweet, they can affect your blood sugar levels. Remember, we are all different, and our bodies will react differently. So you do what allows you to be successful and achieve the results you are looking for.

FOODS TO AVOID

The list of food items to be avoided in IF is a short one. Simply because IF doesn't mean restricting your diet, it means eating everything in moderation. As such, there are no strict food rules in IF, but careful eating during the eating window would ensure maximum benefits for you.

Chips, Cookies, Candies, and Cakes

Bakery items like these contain processed sugar which can cause a rapid rise in blood glucose levels and insulin levels. For this reason, these foods need to be consumed in moderation. Diabetic patients, whether following IF or the standard American diet, need to be more cautious when consuming these items.

The carbohydrates in them create satiety for a few hours, but as soon as the blood sugar level drops, you start feeling hungry just a few hours into fasting. For this reason, eating such items right before the fasting window is not a good idea.

Fruit Drinks

Do you know the composition of a fruit drink? To be labeled "fruit drink," the presence of the following ingredients is a must: fruit juice, added sugar, fruit concentrate, fruit puree, and water. The addition of sugar and food concentrate makes them extremely high in sugar. Fruit juice (citrus fruit juice specifically) is a better option than fruit drinks.

Highly Sweetened Teas and Coffees

The same is valid for sweetened teas and coffees. Even a small cup of sweetened coffee and tea has an extremely high percentage of sugar in it. So while these drinks may offer the same benefits as provided by unsweetened teas and coffees, the sugar present in them is not recommended for a person fasting intermittently.

Sugary Cereals

Sugary cereals that are composed of refined grains and processed sugar are not so good for your health. Such kinds of cereals have incredibly high percentages of sugar, and research has revealed that they can contribute to several chronic diseases like Diabetes and Stroke (Weeratunga et al., 2014). Such cereals make you feel full for a few hours, and then you start craving more carbs, so having sugary cereals during IF is not recommended.

Okay! Let's get to the fun part, i.e., the types of IF methods. You will be amazed to see the diversity of these IF methods. This diversity allows you to choose the best IF method that suits your routine and meal timings.

THE 16/8 TECHNIQUE

The 16/8 technique of IF involves staying in a fasting condition for a total of 16 hours and having an eating window for the rest of the eight hours. During these 16 hours of fasting, drinking water and non-caloric drinks are allowed. This IF method is among those looking to lose weight and attain healthy levels of blood sugar.

The frequency of these fasts ranges from two fasts per week to every day, depending on personal requirements. This method is popular because it has the potential to fit into every lifestyle choice.

How to Do 16/8 Intermittent Fasting?

Initiating a 16/8 IF is easy. All you have to do is figure out an eight-hour eating window, and the rest of the hours will be your fasting time. Following are some popular eating windows for this method:

- 8 a.m. to 4 p.m.
- 9 a.m. to 5 p.m.
- 12 p.m. to 8 p.m.
- 3 a.m. to 11 p.m.

Most people prefer an eating window from 12 p.m. to 8 p.m. since the fasting hours are easier to pass while sleeping, and only breakfast is skipped, allowing you to enjoy complete lunch, snack, and dinner.

The 9 a.m. to 5 p.m. eating window allows you to have a healthy breakfast and a lunch before the fast begins. You can even have a quick snack at 4:30 p.m.

Meal Plan

The meal plan for each style of IF is almost the same, with a few adjustments. The idea for devising a meal plan to follow during the eating window is to include foods with maximum nutritional value. Following a balanced meal plan during the eating hours ensures that the body recovers from the long fasting window and gains energy for the next fasting session.

Nutritionists recommend taking a diet that includes fruits, veggies, whole grains, lean proteins, and healthy fats (like olive oil and avocados).

THE 18/6 TECHNIQUE

The 18/6 IF style is one of the best ones when it comes to shedding extra calories because the fasting window spans a period of 18 hours. The rest of the six hours are set for the eating window. This strategy is also preferred by many because it allows sufficient sleep hours. Besides weight loss, this style is known to achieve high energy levels and a balanced blood sugar level over time. Any form of fasting lasting longer than 12 hours initiates speedy fat burning. This is the reason why 18/6 is an excellent IF method for those looking for a weight loss program.

How to Do 18/6 Intermittent Fasting?

The best time to start on 18/6 IF is between 5:30 p.m. to 6:30 p.m. Eating right before bed is not a good option. This timing will allow you to have lunch around 1:30 p.m. Like other types of IF; you can have water and other calorie-free drinks during your 18 hours of fasting.

Meal Plan

Since the duration of the fasting window is long, your meal plan should contain filling but low-calorie foods.

Below is a list of some highly filling yet low-calorie foods:

- oats
- Greek yogurt (known to decrease calorie consumption in subsequent meals)
- soup
- berries
- eggs (known to reduce the level of hunger hormones)
- chia seeds (labeled superfood due to their nutritional value)
- fish
- cottage cheese
- lean meat
- legumes

THE FAST DIET: 5:2 TECHNIQUE

This is a rather popular form of IF due to its flexibility. 5:2 here refers to days of the week, which means that it includes a five-day period where normal eating is allowed, and the rest of the two days are set for fasting intermittently. In these two days of intermittent fasting, the calorie intake is simply limited to 450-500 calories.

The results of this fasting type have been found to be similar to that of calorie-restriction diets (Hajek et al., 2021).

How to Do 5:2 Intermittent Fasting?

Devising a schedule for 5:2 IF is easy. All you have to do is carefully plan and limit your calorie intake for the two-day fasting period. You can eat whatever you like during the rest of the five days. Generally, the calories on fasting days should be limited to a quarter of what you eat on non-fasting days. This typically translates to 500-700 calories for women.

It is recommended that at least one non-fasting day should be left in between the fasting days. For instance, if you are planning your first fasting day to be Monday, then your second fasting day should be any day between Wednesday to Saturday.

On a fasting day, you can employ any eating pattern, but your ultimate goal should be 500 calories. To achieve this, you could have two complete meals or three small meals with strict calorie measurements.

Meal Plan

There is no single way to eat on fasting days. Several eating patterns have been suggested by the nutritionist, but customized meals can also be planned with the end goal of restricting calories to 25% of the average calorie intake.

Some people eat small meals three times a day. Others start their day with a heavy breakfast and have a light dinner at the end of the day. For others, calorie restrictions mean taking two light meals and skipping the third one entirely.

For people who hardly have time to cook for themselves and rely on fast food, this IF method could provide you with a chance to plan and cook healthy dishes for yourself at least two days a week.

Eating lean proteins can be a great way to start a fasting day. As mentioned before, proteins take hours to digest and thus are a good food choice to get you through the day without feeling hungry. Whitefish, beans, lentils, tofu, eggs, and chicken breast are excellent sources of lean protein.

You also eat berries during your fasting days. Berries of all sorts are rich in good-quality sugars. They can help fulfill your sweet cravings.

EAT, STOP, EAT: 24-HOUR FAST.

The eat-stop-eat is an IF style, which means fasting for 24 hours straight and then continuing on the standard diet until the next 24-hour fast. This fasting style is known for being effective in weight loss, metabolic regulation, and diabetes prevention.

This fasting style appeals to those who find eating with calorie restriction even more difficult. But in reality, going without a meal for 24 hours is not an easy feat. Despite this, several people who are busy during the weekdays and don't have the stamina to go without food for such a long time opt for this style of fasting over the weekends.

How to Do 24-Hour Intermittent Fasting?

Well, that's easy. All you have to do is eat your every day nutritious meals the day before your fasting day. This will provide you the energy to endure hunger on the fasting day. On the fasting day, drinking plenty of water and other non-calorie beverages is recommended. This will keep you hydrated and fresh all day long.

Meal Plan

There is no particular meal plan for the non-fasting days of this style. You just need to eat your normal meals and try to avoid food with too much sugar or fats.

During the fasting day, you should have plenty of fluids to maintain your hydration level. Drinking water mixed with Himalayan salt is highly recommended for this purpose. This salt is loaded with essential minerals and can help in regulating the pH of the body. It also helps to flush out toxins from the body.

WARRIOR DIET I.E. THE 20/4 TECHNIQUE

The 20/4 IF method is also known as the "Warrior Diet" because it was devised by the health and fitness writer Ori Hofmekler, who had experienced the warrior lifestyle while being a part of the Israeli Special Forces. This diet is based on his observations and experiences.

This fasting style reflects the eating pattern of ancient warriors/soldiers who spent most of their day fighting or preparing for fights and only had some time in the evening for a meal. This style is based on the idea that eating meals at the end of the day trains the body to spend the energy in sync with the natural circadian rhythm (sleep-wake cycle).

Warrior Diet may seem a lot like the 16/8 method, but they are pretty different. For one, most of the fasting time in the 16/8 method is spent while sleeping, which makes it very hard to endure. Secondly, the warrior diet allows you to consume about 10% of your daily calories during fasting hours. This IF method has also been linked with reduced belly fat and improved heart health (Stote et al., 2007). According to Ori Hofmekler, adding a workout session to the fasting plan maximizes weight loss and fitness benefits. Don't worry! We will get to the workout options in Chapter 8.

How to Do 20/4 Intermittent Fasting?

This style dictates that 20 hours each day should be spent on minimum caloric intake, and 90% of the calories should be taken in the 4-hour eating windows. However, if you think that a 20-hour long fast is a bit too much to handle, you can adopt one of the modified versions of the warrior plan that allow the consumption of low-calorie drinks and snacks during the fasting windows.

Meal Plan

There are no unique meal plans regarding this fasting style, but eating highly-nutritious meals is recommended during the eating window to maintain your energy level during the fasting session the next day.

Warrior diet is a little lax about caloric intake during the fasting windows. Besides all the non-caloric beverages, you can take vegetables and fruit juices, small amounts of fruits and vegetables, small snacks, vitamins, and supplements.

ONE MEAL A DAY OMAD: THE 23/1 TECHNIQUE

One Meal a Day Diet is a technique that is one of the most intense and difficult-to-follow plans that includes fasting for almost 23 hours in a day and eating all the calories in just one hour.

This technique is one of the best when it comes to losing body fats. The idea is to push the body to use all of the extra body fats to derive energy. After almost 12 hours of fasting, the body starts burning fats, and this continues for the next 10 to 11 hours before the eating window starts. This method has shown promising results when it comes to weight loss. 10 to 12 weeks of OMAD can help you shed 7 to 11 pounds. The OMAD plan is ideal for people diagnosed with pre-diabetes and the risk of heart disease. While this plan may produce quick results, it is not easy to sustain those results. People who follow this plan stop abruptly as soon as they start seeing positive results. Such people tell themselves that they have done enough fasting and that they should eat to "reward" this effort. This results in abrupt weight gain and reversal of all the positive effects.

How to Do OMAD Intermittent Fasting?

The OMAD plan does not dictate your eating hour. You can pick any time that suits you, eat till you are full, and start your fast. After you have done so, get yourself busy and never stop to think of a meal for the next 23 hours. Proponents of this fasting style say that this method is very effective when it comes to elevating energy levels or attention span. For diabetic patients, this plan can lead to greater control over blood glucose levels (Arnason et al., 2017).

This IF technique should be carried out in sessions of 5-7 days. There should be 3 to 4 recovery days between these sessions.

Meal Plan

The perks offered by the OMAD plan is that you can eat anything you like in that one-hour eating window, but since the time is limited before your next fast begins, you cannot just eat junk food during that one hour. You have to incorporate nutritious yet filling foods in your diet to gear you up for your next fast.

ALTERNATE DAY FASTING (ADF)

The IF plan is the one where you fast one day and eat normally the next day. This fasting style efficiently cuts your caloric intake in half. It is easier to stick to. Combining ADF with exercise doubles its weight loss and muscle gain benefits.

How to Do Alternate Day Fasting?

Regarding the execution of ADF, there are two opinions. One advocates fasting entirely on the fasting days, while the other suggests consuming 25% of the normal caloric intake on the fasting days. Consuming a few calories during the fast shows better results in that it makes the fast easy to endure, and the hunger hormone's production remains unaffected.

Meal Plan

The meal plan to be followed in this IF method is simple. Eat your regular meals on the non-fasting days, and if you are choosing to consume 25% of calories on the fasting day, then all you have to do is devise a plan that can help you restrict your calories to the said 25%.

You can do this by eating two small meals during the fast or taking a single meal. You can continue to drink calorie-free drinks on fasting days.

Some healthy, low-caloric food ideas that are below 500 calories are

- 4 to 5 boiled eggs and 3 cups of soup.
- 1 to 2 cups of Greek yogurt with berries.
- 3 to 4 ounces of salad with any lean meat dish of your choice.

SPONTANEOUS MEAL SKIPPING

Spontaneous meal skipping is the easiest and most popular IF technique. Everyone misses a meal here and there, and this is precisely what the Spontaneous Meal Skipping method is. Some people do it because they are working late and have to skip meals; others do it because they are feeling too tired to cook a meal for themselves. There isn't much scientific research regarding the efficacy of Spontaneous

Meal Skipping but abandoning 600 to 1000-calorie meals four to five times a month would surely have a positive health impact.

CIRCADIAN RHYTHM FASTING

Circadian Rhythm Fasting (CRF) is a type of fasting that has an eating window between the early few hours of the day. Experts suggest that this eating window should be between 8 a.m. to 6 p.m. This means that the best hours for fasting are from 6 p.m. to 8 a.m.

The idea behind this method is to synchronize the cycles of hormone production with nutrition. Circadian rhythms are the daily cycles driven by the brain with input from several physical conditions of the body. Several studies promote the efficacy of this IF style. Circadian Rhythm Fasting is an umbrella term that includes both time-restricted fasting and alternate-day fasting, but the basic concept is to restrict the caloric intake to a specific time during the day. This method has shown beneficial results in animal models in terms of metabolic improvement and the prevention of chronic diseases (Longo & Panda, 2016).

How to Do Circadian Rhythm Fasting?

The best time to start CRF is late afternoon. By this time, you should have eaten your fill and should be ready to begin your fast.

Meal Plan

Again, there are no specific meal requirements in a Circadian Rhythm Fast. You can eat everything you like. It is the timing of your meals that matters. Since mealtime is the same every day, you won't have to go hungry for a full day. Getting 7-8 hours of sleep and working out is recommended to maximize the benefits of Circadian Rhythm Fasting.

EXTENDED FASTING OR PROLONGED FASTING

It is a fasting style that involves fasting for 36 hours or more. Fasting for 36-48 hours is nothing new. People have fasted for this duration in the past. The reason why this extreme form of fasting is getting popular is the fact that research has revealed its benefits for most people. This fasting style is tough to adopt and maintain. However, one study indicates that this fasting method can be viable for extremely obese individuals. During this study, an obese person with 456 pounds of weight fasted for 382 days and ended up losing 276 pounds (Stewart & Fleming, 1973).

How to Do Extended Intermittent Fasting?

This form of IF targets your metabolism and energy levels. Extended period without food pushes your system to run without glucose and use fat as the primary energy source. For this fasting style, all you need to do is fill yourself up with as much as you can eat at mealtime, say at dinner and then fast for the next day completely. You can take a zero-calorie drink during the fast. On the second of your fast, you can decide if you want to fast for precisely 36 hours or do you have the stamina to *extend* your fast even more. You can prolong your fast up to 48 hours at max.

Meal Plan

After your fasting hours are complete, make sure that you start eating gradually and at intervals. Introducing food at a rapid pace could overstimulate your gut and lead to bloating, diarrhea and nausea. Therefore, your first meal should be a light snack. You can take a smoothie or a light salad at the start. After two to three hours, you can have a proper meal. On non-fasting days, you can eat your regular meals without consuming too many calorie-high foods.

For safety reasons, this fasting style should only be employed once or twice a month. I think you have got a clear idea about each of these IF methods. If not, go through them again and decide which IF plan suits you the most.

Celebrity Success Stories

Spanish star Elsa Pataky started intermittent fasting back in 2019 when her husband, Chris Hemsworth, introduced it to her. In the beginning, she had doubts regarding the efficacy of this style, but gradually she started noticing the positive changes in her body and energy levels. She started to read more about IF and now views it as the best anti-aging and weight loss method.

The Lesley Leach Program

If the 16/8 method is your preferred IF style, you need to train your body to endure hunger for those 16 hours, and for that, you need practice. Our bodies are conditioned for food with a gap of two hours, but we can increase this gap. Starting with 16/8 IF is easy. As I mentioned earlier, all you need to do is figure out your eight-hour eating window. For instance, If you start eating at 8 a.m., stop eating at 4 p.m. and start your fast. If you start eating at 1 p.m., stop eating at 9 p.m. and start your fast.

Given below is a 28-day fasting planner for you. You use it to track your progress with this fasting planner. All you need is to log the hours that you spent in the eating window and your fasting window. Based on the duration of your fast, you can rate your performance.

My 16/8 IF performance	**Day 1**	**Day 2**	**Day 3**	**Day 4**	**Day 5**	**Day 6**	**Day 7**
Started eating at							
Stopped eating at							
Fasted for							
Performance rating							

My 16/8 IF performance	Day 8	Day 9	Day 10	Day 11	Day 12	Day 13	Day 14
Started eating at							
Stopped eating at							
Fasted for							
Performance rating							

My 16/8 IF performance	Day 15	Day 16	Day 17	Day 18	Day 19	Day 20	Day 21
Started eating at							
Stopped eating at							
Fasted for							
Performance rating							

My 16/8 IF performance	Day 22	Day 23	Day 24	Day 25	Day 26	Day 27	Day 28
Started eating at							
Stopped eating at							
Fasted for							
Performance rating							

You can rate your performance out of three stars:

Three stars - I fasted for 16 hours or more

Two stars - I fasted for 12-16 hours

One star - I fasted for less than 12 hours

3

INTERMITTENT FASTING FOR WOMEN: WHAT'S IN IT FOR YOU?

The differences in the height, weight, physique, and stamina of men and women mean differences in their response to IF. The basic difference between them is the working and regulation of their reproductive systems. For women, this system operates in cycles, and the menstrual phase of this cycle requires a little care. To do IF comfortably during the menstrual phase, staying hydrated and eating lots of leafy greens can help deal with menstrual cramps and headaches.

There are several age-related issues that contribute to weight gain in women. The major being that as we age, our metabolism slows down, yet our appetites have not. That's where IF comes in. It increases our metabolism and lowers the risk of several age-related problems.

WHY WOMEN SHOULD DO INTERMITTENT FASTING?

Let's have a look at how IF proves beneficial for women.

Heart Health

Problems like high blood pressure and high cholesterol levels may not be common in young women. Still, with age, these problems start appearing primarily for the reasons that women become less active with age, their eating habits get less healthy, they hardly have time to cook for themselves, and they have even less time to exercise. All of these unhealthy lifestyle choices, when combined with declining health, can lead to heart issues.

IF has proved efficient in improving the heart health of women and men alike. Varady et al. (2013) studied the effects of alternate-day fasting (ADF) on 32 normal and overweight subjects. The study reported a positive decline in blood pressure of 30 subjects who completed the 12-week trial. A decrease in the plasma concentrations of triglycerides and LDL was also reported.

Diabetes

We have previously discussed how IF helps regulate blood sugar levels and increase sensitivity toward insulin.

Most of us have trained our bodies to digest and metabolize nutrients every two hours because that's how often some of us eat. This gives our bodies a lot to deal with; a lot of glucose needs to be metabolized and stored. Normally, our bodies manage that by producing insulin that ultimately regulates glucose levels. But with increasing age and declining organ function, such high glucose levels lead to problems. Diabetes is one such problem when the body fails to regulate blood glucose levels. In Diabetes (type 2), either the body stops making sufficient insulin or the body cells become unresponsive to insulin.

IF has been shown to deal with prediabetes and lower the risk of type 2 diabetes in general. Harvie et al. (2010) reported that six months of IF showed a 29% reduction in insulin levels which ultimately decreased insulin resistance by 19% in 100 overweight and obese women.

Weight Loss

IF is highly effective when it comes to losing extra pounds. Short-term but periodic fasting can help you lose weight without causing any side effects. For weight loss, IF is as effective as calorie restriction diets. Although long-term weight loss effects need to be studied, IF has proved effective in causing short-term fat burning by up to 3-8% over a duration of 3-24 weeks (Barnosky et al., 2014).

Total Caloric Reduction

IF has also been found to lower overall calorie intake, meaning that allotting a specific time for eating causes people to consume fewer calories than they would typically consume. There is no clear reason as to why this happens, but when faced with the given choice to eat more in less time, people tend to eat less.

Johnstone et al. (2002) reported that on a typical day following a 36-hour fast, people found it hard to eat more than their normal capacity. And even when they ate extra, a drop of 1900 calories in their diet was recorded.

Reduced Inflammation

Inflammation occurs every time our bodies try to fight an infection or injury. To achieve this, several mechanisms are employed, and while that's happening, we may experience several symptoms, including fever, fatigue, abdominal and chest pain, joint pain, mouth sores, and skin rashes.

If these symptoms occur for a few days, we call it acute inflammation, but if they occur for several months to years, we categorize it under chronic inflammation. Chronic inflammation occurs when the infection or injury is too big for the body to handle. Chronic inflammation is also a leading cause of diabetes, heart disease, joint disease, and several types of allergies.

Research has revealed that prolonged IF lessens chronic inflammation and as well the risk of cardiac diseases.

Improved Psychological Well-Being

Weight management is a serious issue for many people in their 50s and a cause for their unhappiness and negative body image. IF deals effectively with this issue as well. People who fast intermittently tend to have a positive mindset for several reasons. One, IF improves their mood and energy levels, and second, it helps manage their weight which leads to a positive body image. All of this contributes to their psychological well-being.

Increased Longevity

The case of increased lifespan through IF has been proved for several animal models such as mice, rats, and fish. Inferring data from these experiments, we can conclude that IF has the same effects on humans. This is because IF reduces the risk of several chronic diseases.

Preserve Muscle Mass

Muscle loss is a common problem in people in their 50s. IF is known to increase the production of Human Growth Hormone (HGH), which in turn promotes muscle building. Meanwhile, other hormones like the hunger hormone (Ghrelin) act to prevent muscle wasting.

BENEFITS

In recent times, most women have turned to IF to reduce the risk or reverse the symptoms of three health problems: cancer, Polycystic Ovary Syndrome (PCOS), and diabetes. Let's see how that happens.

Cancer and Fasting

Over the last few decades, the prevalence of cancer has increased manifolds. This may be due to rising levels of pollution or our unhealthy food choices and recurring infections.

Research suggests that IF proves extremely valuable when it comes to lowering cancer risk, lowering cancer-related symptoms, and improving the efficacy of anticancer therapies. Several theories have been presented over time to explain these effects.

- Our bodies are constantly subjected to stress (oxidative stress). This stress may be due to smoking, alcohol consumption, unhealthy food, and level of activity. With increasing age, oxidative stress increases the risk of cancer. IF is known to lower this oxidative stress by providing the cells with sufficient time to rest and cleanse themselves.

- Cancer develops when the regulatory system in a cell goes haywire. Old body cells are more prone to developing cancer than new ones. And this is where IF comes to the rescue. Staying hungry for several hours initiates autophagy, which gets rid of old and disease-prone cells, thus reducing the cancer risk.
- IF reduces cancer risk by preventing major chronic disorders that may lead to cancer development. These disorders include type 2 diabetes and obesity.
- IF is also known to boost the production of immune cells and refuel the immune system to produce more tumor-killing cells.
- Since tumor cells have high metabolic activity going on in them, they require more energy and more glucose. But the lowering of glucose levels during IF cuts down that glucose supply, and so tumor growth is slowed down.
- Lack of energy supply to tumor cells makes them a better target for chemotherapy and other tumor-killing procedures while protecting normal body cells.
- IF boosts the production of stem cells. These are the cells that act as raw materials for the body to form new body cells. These stem cells are extremely vital during cancer patients' recovery and rehabilitation.

They reduce inflammation and provide relief during cancer recovery.

For people looking to lower cancer risk through IF, nutritionists recommend avoiding red meat, alcohol, and processed food. However, cancer patients are advised to seek medical advice before trying IF. Provision of a nutrient-rich diet, maintenance of appropriate hydration levels, and preservation of muscle mass should be the number one priority for cancer patients. Therefore, extreme fasting styles with longer fasting windows are not recommended for them.

PCOS and Intermittent Fasting

PCOS is a common hormonal disorder in women that affects women of childbearing age. There are several symptoms of PCOS, including:

- irregular or non-existent menstruation
- Obesity
- infertility issues
- cysts on ovaries
- acne
- excessive hair loss or hair growth (on the face and chest)
- mood swings
- Depression

- insulin resistance

Insulin resistance means that the body is unlikely to respond properly to insulin levels in the body, which will lead to poorly managed blood glucose levels, and this means a higher risk of type 2 diabetes and obesity. Lack of hormonal management leads to higher levels of hormones like androgen in the blood, which then leads to fertility issues, mood swings, acne, and excessive hair growth.

Fortunately, all of these issues can be solved through dietary and lifestyle interventions, and this is where IF comes in. The research in this area is thin, but preliminary data suggest that IF could help women with PCOS by lowering their insulin resistance and androgen levels (Chiofalo et al., 2017).

Let's see how IF can help with PCOS:

- Calorie reduction that occurs as a result of IF could help in weight management for PCOS-affected women.
- A decrease in blood glucose levels could help lower insulin production, and this could improve insulin sensitivity.
- IF could help manage the level of hormones that trigger mood swings and excessive hair growth.
- IF could help lower PCOS-induced inflammation.

In some cases, IF can worsen PCOS symptoms. For instance, excessive eating during the eating window could increase the stress on insulin production, and insulin resistance could get worse. For women with eating disorders, shifting to an extreme IF method could lead to unregulated eating patterns. In such cases, working with a nutritionist can help you design a customized IF plan for you.

Type 2 Diabetes and Intermittent Fasting

We have discussed how IF helps people diagnosed with prediabetes and lowers their diabetes risk through the regulation of blood glucose, improvement of insulin sensitivity, and management of their weight. But all of these things are important for diabetic patients too.

Let's see how diabetic patients can benefit from IF.

Research suggests that IF can lower insulin resistance in diabetic patients (Rohner et al., 2021). It is also thought that weight loss achieved through IF could also help improve insulin sensitivity in type 2 diabetes patients.

However, some experts are of the view that IF can have a negative impact on people whose glucose regulation is already stunted. According to them, such long intervals between meals can cause poor blood glucose levels, which can ultimately cause fatigue. Restricting meal time to a few hours can cause people to make unhealthy food choices, which will impact their weight and glucose level. For diabetic patients, a rapid fall in their glucose level could lead to a condition called hypoglycemia. This could lead to issues like dizziness, nausea, blurred vision, and rapid heartbeat. Contrastingly, a rapid rise in sugar level after an eating window could lead to hyperglycemia, which increases the risk of nerve damage, kidney damage, stroke, and eye-related disorders.

Owing to these circumstances, it is preferred that diabetic individuals should fast intermittently only after getting clearance from their medical supervisor or nutritionist. It is recommended that diabetic patients should opt for short fasting hours to sustain their glucose level within the normal range.

HOW TO SUCCEED WITH IF?

Most people, when picking an IF method, think they have the energy and stamina to begin their IF with a bigger fasting duration, but this could prove challenging for their bodies. You see, human bodies are unable to adapt to sudden changes. For instance, a body trained for three meals and several snack times could get overwhelmed when subjected to a 20/4 method. Therefore, to ensure success with IF, a slow and steady approach is required. Here is how this can be done:

1. Figure the most effortless fasting style for yourself. Keep your medical history, current health status,

activity level, and eating habits in mind while you do so. For most women over 50s, the 5:2 IF method is recommended as it involves only two days of calorie restriction. You can slowly progress to methods with longer fasting windows.

2. Your hydration levels can determine you're IF success rate. Maintaining a high hydration level will lower the side effects of fasting. Taking lots of fluids during your fast will ensure that you stay energized and have something to put in your stomach throughout that period. The color of your urine is a good indicator of your hydration level. It should always be light yellow in color.
3. Our digestive system is designed to release digestive juices during our usual eating hours, and this makes us crave food even more. Keeping yourself busy, especially during these hours, will take your mind off your hunger.
4. Make sure that the foods you are consuming during the eating window are nutrient-dense to help you regain your strength and energy. Excessive consumption of processed foods is not recommended; however, if you feel that your body responds well to such food items, you can consume them in moderation.

Following the above-mentioned tips will make your fasting time easier, and you will be able to incorporate IF into your normal routine.

IS IF SAFE?

The question regarding the safety and viability of IF is an important one. While IF may prove beneficial for most people belonging to all ages and genders and for several body conditions, some people should not fast intermittently, and even if they do, they should do so under medical supervision to proceed safely.

According to the experts, people who should consult with a healthcare professional before fasting intermittently are:

Children and tweens

The part of the brain that controls our hunger and tells us to eat is not so developed in children. This is the reason why children often skip meals when the food is not to their liking or if they are too busy with some activity. At other times, they may binge eat, especially if they get their hands on fast food. IF can promote these binging habits, so it is better if children refrain from IF. They should be encouraged to eat healthy, nutrient-rich meals three times a day.

Pregnant women

Pregnancy is a period that requires women to consume extra calories to support fetal development. Therefore, pregnancy is not the perfect time to cut calories. IF can cause severe nutritional deficiency during pregnancy and lead to the infant's stunted growth.

Women who are breastfeeding

IF is known to interfere with the normal calorie intake, hormonal balance, and energy levels of an individual. All of these parameters also affect the production of milk in breastfeeding mothers. For this reason, IF is not recommended for such ladies.

Diabetes type 1 patient

Diabetes type 1 is a disorder where the normal production of insulin is low. Diabetes type 1 patients need to take insulin to meet the demand. They also require a constant energy supply in the form of calories to maintain their normal sugar levels. While research shows that Type 2 Diabetes patients can fast intermittently, no such data has been collected for Type 1 patients. Regarding these patients, there is a concern that they can develop hypoglycemia during long periods of fasting.

People suffering from eating disorders and psychological issues

IF can create health complications for individuals with eating disorders. For overweight individuals, a sudden withdrawal can have a rebound effect which can cause them to consume more calories than before. For already underweight individuals, IF can further create nutritional imbalance and be life-threatening. Similarly, if you are having a hard time regulating your mood, you should seek the help of a medical professional. Calorie intake is linked to mood regulation, so in the absence of food for most of the day, you can suffer anxiety and depression.

People who start developing serious side effects every time they try IF

People who try IF and develop severe side effects are advised to refrain from IF. Such individuals are advised to talk to their doctor to see if they can help minimize these side effects, but if these effects persist, they should abandon fasting.

IF and Menstrual Cycle

We have previously seen how women's bodies respond differently to IF than men's. The reason behind this difference is that their reproductive systems operate differently. For women's bodies, it is a monthly cycle of menstruation that causes fluctuation in their hormonal levels, and it determines how they respond to IF. Hormonal changes during each month are known to cause instability in their energy and stress levels as well. For this reason, women need care when trying IF.

During the menstruation phase especially, the stress response is heightened, and energy levels may be low; this can make IF hard. Additionally, there is bloating, constipation, and pain in the back and stomach that doesn't make IF any easier. Also, in the week before menstruation, the hormonal stress is so high that adding an extra stressor like IF could prove problematic for some.

Therefore, experts recommend taking a balanced approach for women when deciding on the IF plan. IF should be adjusted for different phases of the cycle. For this, take note of how you are feeling at different times of the month, what IF window you are following as well as results you make be looking for. If your goal is true weight loss, know that your body weight will be altered at certain times of the month. If you are one who weighs yourself often, don't get discouraged by the number. If things get bothersome, talk to your healthcare provider is advised.

Safety Levels of IF

So far, IF has been found safe and beneficial for most women; however, owing to their sensitive hormonal issues and complicated monthly cycle, it is advised that women should apply a different approach than men. To ensure that IF is safe and effective, women should follow these tips:

- Avoid fasting on consecutive days, especially when trying extreme forms of IF.
- Avoid extreme workout sessions on fasting days, especially during the last few hours of your fast.

- Eat nutrient-rich foods during the eating window to fuel your body and maintain hormonal balance.
- Always start with easy fasting methods and periodically move to more demanding IF methods, but only if you still feel you have the stamina to do so.
- Switch back to a low-intensity IF plan if you start developing serious side effects like period irregularity, digestive issues, and skin and hair problems.
- Consult with a healthcare provider and proceed with caution if you are trying to conceive. IF could disturb the normal levels of sex hormones which can hurt your chances of conceiving.

IF and Menopause

Menopause is a period where metabolic and hormonal fluctuations in the woman's body cause several undesirable changes to normal body functioning. Lowering levels of certain hormones can also lead to weight gain, muscle loss, and inflammation.

Fortunately, IF has been found effective in dealing with all of these issues. The metabolic regulation achieved through IF could help lower that stubborn belly fat (Varady et al., 2021). This could also balance stress-related hormones. The combined effect of IF and working out can help deal with muscle loss and inflammation. It has been found that except for a few cases where women are sensitive to diet changes IF is generally safe and beneficial for menopausal women.

Celebrity Success Stories

Fifty-year-old American actress Jennifer Aniston is all praise for IF. She shared her IF lifestyle in a magazine interview in October 2019. She revealed that IF makes her look and feel good.

She follows the 16/8 IF method. Talking about her IF plan, she said that she fasts during the first part of the day while her eating window is set for the evening. During the fasting window, she relies on liquids like celery juice and coffee.

The Lesley Leach Program

For the eat-stop-eat IF method, you need to make sure there is a 22 to 24 hours gap between your meals. On a non-fasting day, eat normally, then start counting your fasting hours from your last meal of that day. Skip the next two meals and eat only when you have fasted for 22 to 24 hours.

For instance:

If you start your fast from lunch on the previous day, you will skip dinner and breakfast and have lunch after 22 to 24 hours have passed. You don't have to be strict about completing 24 hours of fasting. A relaxation of 1 to 2 hours is allowed.

Given below is a 28-day fasting planner for your 24-hour IF. You use it to track your progress with this fasting planner. For starters, you can mark each day as either normal or fasting. If it's a normal day, note down your meal times and if it's a fasting day, note the timing of your first meal when you break your fast. Lastly, note the duration of your fast and how you feel after fasting for that duration. How you feel mentally and physically after 24-hour long fasts will help you determine whether this method suits you or not.

My IF performance	Day 1	Day 2	Day 3	Day 4	Day 5	Day 6	Day 7
Normal or Fasting Day?							
Breakfast time							
Lunchtime							
Dinner time							
Did I fast for 22-24 hrs?							
How do I feel after the fast?							

My IF performance	Day 8	Day 9	Day 10	Day 11	Day 12	Day 13	Day 14
Normal or Fasting Day?							
Breakfast time							
Lunchtime							
Dinner time							
Did I fast for 22-24 hrs?							
How do I feel after the fast?							

My IF performance	Day 15	Day 16	Day 17	Day 18	Day 19	Day 20	Day 21
Normal or Fasting Day?							
Breakfast time							
Lunchtime							
Dinner time							
Did I fast for 22-24 hrs?							
How do I feel after the fast?							

My IF performance	Day 22	Day 23	Day 24	Day 25	Day 26	Day 27	Day 28
Normal or Fasting Day?							
Breakfast time							
Lunchtime							
Dinner time							
Did I fast for 22-24 hrs?							
How do I feel after the fast?							

4

OVER 50 LIFESTYLE AND INTERMITTENT FASTING

Reaching the second half of a century is undoubtedly an achievement in one's life. This half-a-century brings with it experience, wisdom, and a new zest for life. This is also a time of great biological changes, which are more pronounced in the case of women. These changes are collectively termed menopause.

Menopause is defined as a 12-month period after a women's last menstruation. The period leading up to this point is called perimenopause or menopausal transition, and this period is characterized by gradual changes in the menstrual cycle, hot flashes, and hormonal changes. Perimenopause can start between the ages of 45 to 55 and usually lasts for seven to fourteen years. This is a period of great biological and physical changes. The metabolism slows down, fat cells start storing more fats, sex hormones decrease, and bones stop storing calcium. All of these changes mean that menopause is a time when our bodies are prone to gaining weight, and bones are likely to get brittle. This also means that you will experience changes in your brain and heart activity which will ultimately affect your energy levels and brain activity.

MENOPAUSE WEIGHT GAIN AND IF

The changes occurring slowly during perimenopause are completed during menopause; once these changes are completed, the body enters the post-menopausal stage. This is the period where women are most vulnerable to bone disorders, weight gain, heart disease, and muscle loss.

Let's see what leads to this vulnerability.

Causes of Menopausal Weight Gain

Before menopause, women are likely to gain more fat around their thighs, but after menopause, this fat distribution is changed. Menopausal women are more likely to have fat around their bellies. The reason for this change is not known for sure, but the drop in the female sex hormone estrogen is most likely responsible for this change. Besides hormonal change, other risk factors that influence weight gain after menopause are age, diet, activity level, and family history.

Age is an important risk factor because, with age, people tend to get less active owing to muscle loss and fatigue. This contributes to weight gain. Among all of the risk factors for weight gain, diet and activity levels can be adjusted to ensure effective weight management. This also means that after menopause, weight management is solely dependent on personal choices. Making healthy food choices and incorporating exercise in your daily routine can ensure that your weight is kept within a normal range.

Weight gain during menopause can become difficult to shed, and this can have serious health implications later in life. Extra fats, especially those around the midsection, can lead to problems like type 2 diabetes, breathing problems, and heart disorders.

Causes of Menopausal Muscle Loss

Again, the decreasing levels of estrogen after menopause are implicated in muscle loss in women. The exact mechanism for this is not known for sure, but the absence of this hormone increases the loss of muscle fibers' quality and amount. Factors that increase the risk of muscle deterioration are lack of exercise, alcohol consumption, and a protein-deficient diet.

The best strategy to deal with muscle loss is eating a protein-rich diet and following an exercise routine that targets the major muscle groups; legs, back, chest, biceps, triceps, shoulders, and abdominals.

Causes of Menopausal Bones Weakness

Dips in estrogen levels are also the leading cause of bone weakness in women over 50s. This hormone also regulates calcium storage in the bones, and when that decreases, bones start getting brittle. This puts women at a greater risk of developing bone fractures.

Other risk factors that affect bone health are activity, smoking, alcohol consumption, and diet. This suggests that even in the absence of estrogen hormone, a carefully planned regimen of exercise and diet can make sure that the bones maintain this strength.

Causes of Menopausal Brain Changes

Menopause affects not just the reproductive system of women; it affects their brains too. These effects can be both direct and indirect. For one, falling estrogen levels alter the brain's capacity to consume glucose, which ultimately leads the brain to slow down.

Falling estrogen levels don't allow complete activation of the hypothalamus (the part implicated in temperature regulation), leading women to suffer hot flashes during menopause. Insufficient activation of the sleep-wake region of the brain causes sleep issues. The memory center suffers as well. Lastly, rapid fluctuations in estrogen levels cause mood swings in women going through menopause. This may lead to anxiety, depression, anger, and a negative self-image. When it comes to anxiety disorders, women in their 50s make up the greatest risk group (Remes et al., 2016).

Manage Your Menopause

The hormonal changes that women go through during menopause weigh heavily on their overall health. But even when these changes can't be reversed, sticking to a basic weight management plan can help keep things from getting worse.

Be Active

Maintaining an active lifestyle is vital for a lot of reasons. First, this can help you stay energized and prevent your body from developing mobility issues. For this reason, people with disorders like arthritis are advised to include exercise in their routine. Secondly, incorporating a carefully designed routine of aerobic exercise and strength training can help you build muscle or at least prevent muscle deterioration. Muscle building also makes weight loss more effortless as the process of muscle building consumes extra calories and burns fat.

Aerobic activities like brisk walking or jogging sessions are also helpful in reducing stress and improving brain function

(Sharma et al., 2006). These activities can also reduce the risk of chronic disorders. Experts recommend aerobic exercise for at least two hours every week, and strength training exercises are recommended at least twice a week for the effective management of menopause-related issues.

Keep Your Calories In Check

A significant calorie reduction is required for women in their 50s to ensure the maintenance of a healthy weight. For this purpose, several diets like the vegan diet and low-carb diet are recommended, but the best way to restrict calories is to consume foods that are low in calories or to adopt an eating pattern (like IF) that naturally limits the calories. Low-calorie foods include leafy greens, lean proteins, beans, legumes, and fruits. Also, limiting the intake of red meat, dairy products, and processed food can help lower the overall calories.

Limit Your Sugar Intake

There are some foods and drinks that may not provide so many nutrients but are ridiculously high in added sugars. This makes them extremely loaded with calories. These include soft drinks, juices, energy drinks, ice cream, cakes, cookies, and pies.

Limiting such items in your diet can help cut extra calories, which can shed extra weight on your body.

Limit Alcohol Consumption

Alcohol consumption ramps up your overall calorie intake and contributes to heart problems, obesity, and diabetes. So, limiting alcohol consumption is always a good step towards a healthy lifestyle.

Seek Help Whenever Required

The changes during menopause are sometimes so overwhelming that dealing with them seems impossible, but if you are someone who is committed to lifestyle adjustments, you can consult with a healthcare professional for technical support. Your family and friends can be your emotional support during the whole process. Having someone who is going through the same process is even better. This way will have a companion for encouragement and support.

How Menopausal Women Can Benefit From IF?

IF is an all-in-one deal, it is an effective method that keeps a check on calorie intake, holds the threat of chronic diseases at bay, and provides a boost to mental health and physical fitness.

To Prevent Weight Gain

There are several methods through which IF prevents weight gain in women over 50. First, IF helps balance hormone levels. Balancing the hormone levels lowers the chances of fat accumulation in the belly. Secondly, giving long breaks between meals allows the body to modulate insulin levels. This increases the body's sensitivity towards insulin as well as enables the body to use extra fat to derive energy. A dip in insulin boosts HGH production, which helps to build muscles. These newly gained muscles improve metabolism, which boosts fat burning. Having limited eating windows instill mindful eating habits, thus lowering your chances of consuming fatty foods, added sugars, and unhealthy snacks.

All of these processes work collaboratively to prevent weight gain.

To Boost Mental Health

IF provides a balance to the rapidly fluctuating hormones in menopausal women. This occurs due to a drop in blood sugar levels which are known to cause stress and anxiety. The body and brain get the much-needed rest, and this creates a sense of calm.

Fluctuating glucose levels which were previously creating brain fog, are lessened, and this improves energy and focus.

To Promote Heart Health

High blood pressure is a common issue among women after menopause. This is also a leading cause of heart-related disorders. IF proves beneficial here as well by reducing blood pressure and reducing bad cholesterol in the blood vessels. The reduction in the blood levels of two important items, i.e., triglycerides and low-density lipoproteins, lowers the risk of cardiovascular disorders (CVD). On the other hand, long intervals in the intake of important nutrients help to regulate blood pressure during intermittent fasting.

To Boost Bone Health and Muscle Gain

The chaos created by falling estrogen levels is handled well by IF. IF promotes the production of hormones that help improve bone strength. It also helps in building muscles by promoting HGH production. Eating a protein-rich diet and doing strength training prevents muscle wasting and allows you to retain those muscles, both during and after menopause.

To Promote Gut Health

Falling estrogen levels disturb the digestive processes as well. This means that more time is required for the food to pass along the system. IF deals effectively with these issues too. First, the long breaks between meals allow sufficient time for proper digestion of the one meal before the next meal arrives. Extra consumption of fluids during the fasting window deals with the constipation issue too. Giving long breaks between meals allows sufficient time for the stomach and intestinal lining to repair.

What Makes IF the Best Weight Loss Plan?

Compared to other calories restricting diets, IF is a natural weight loss plan which does not involve strict calorie calculations. It reduces total caloric intake naturally by implementing a system of eating windows. In contrast to the dieting regimens, IF not only limits calories but also promotes excess fat burning. Unlike strict diets that may cause rebound weight gain, IF is an easy weight loss plan that's simple and entails no specific dietary restrictions.

IF is also known to produce quick results because, in IF, we have both calorie reduction and fat burning that work together to lower your body weight.

5 Intermittent Fasting Tips

Figure Out the Best IF Method

This is something that you have to decide on your own. You have to figure out the method that works best for your body. For this purpose, you can try different fasting windows and various fasting durations until you find the best fit. However, if you are currently under the care of a doctor, I recommend consulting with them. They can help you with the IF plan selection.

Pay Attention to How Your Body Responds to IF

The best scale to gauge your performance during IF is to listen to your body and how it responds during and after the fast. If you start feeling hungry a few hours into the fast, you need to incorporate more proteins into your diet (they take more time to digest). However, if you feel that your body is responding well to IF, your hunger is under control, and you are performing well throughout the day, that means your body is showing a positive response to your IF schedule.

Don't Quit, Deal With the Side Effects of IF

Some people quit IF as soon as they start experiencing minor discomfort. I know IF is not an easy feat, especially not at the start when your body is not familiar with the fasting schedule. But instead of quitting, you should give your body some time to adjust. Simply doing that will resolve minor side effects like nausea, headache, and irritability; your stomach might need some more time to adjust.

Avoid Overeating

Overeating during the eating windows can sabotage the efforts that you put in during fasting hours. Not only that, but overeating during these hours can cause digestive issues as well. To avoid that, make sure you eat enough to gear you up for the next fasting session.

Be Realistic With Your Goals

IF is a proven method that can help you attain your ideal weight, but it's not magic. You will have to work slowly and consistently to achieve your ideal fitness level with IF. to ensure that you need to set realistic goals that can encourage and motivate you throughout the journey.

EFFICACY OF IF FOR WOMEN OVER 50

There is a huge amount of research data that suggests that IF is highly effective for both premenopausal and post-menopausal women. One study reported that the level of bad cholesterol dropped more in postmenopausal women than in premenopausal women following alternate-day fasting (ADF). Fat mass, blood sugar, blood pressure, and insulin resistance showed an equal drop for both premenopausal and postmenopausal women (Lin et al., 2020).

Another study that looked at the impact of fasting for 18 to 20 hours a day showed similar results for obese women regardless of their menopausal status. All of these women showed weight loss and positive metabolic changes (Cienfuegos et al., 2021).

These studies indicate that women over 50 have more to gain from IF. Owing to an apparent decline in the sex hormone levels in these women, they are at a higher risk of obesity, heart disorders, and other chronic diseases. And this makes them an even better candidate for IF than premenopausal women.

7 FASTING TIPS WHEN YOU'RE OVER 50

If you are new to IF, follow the tips below to make your IF journey smooth and easy.

Start With an Easy Plan

When I first started IF, I was a voracious eater. I used to have at least three complete meals and snacks throughout the eating window. So, when I switched to IF, 18/6 plan, I found myself struggling with hunger. I figured I had started with a hard plan. Then, I revised my IF plan and reduced my fasting hours to 9-10 hours a day. There were overnight hours, and s0, most of my fasting hours were spent sleeping. Gradually, I widened my fasting window and was able to resume my original 16/8 plan within one month.

Get Enough Calories

People who are new to intermittent fasting either end up consuming too much during the eating windows or fail to consume sufficient calories that are necessary to ensure the refueling of their bodies. Consuming a balanced amount of nutrients is essential to ensure IF success.

Prioritize Protein

The importance of proteins for women over 50 can never be overemphasized. The provision of proteins ensures that the body has sufficient fuel to rebuild muscles and reverse the muscle lost during menopause. To address this, experts recommend the consumption of foods high in proteins, including lean meat, fish, legumes, lentils, Greek yogurt, tofu, etc.

Do Strength Training

All forms of exercise are known to act complementary to IF by promoting an early fat-burning process, but strength training promotes muscle building as well. Strength training creates small cuts or tears in the muscle fibers, and this initiates a process of muscle repair and renewal.

This process is extremely important for women over 50s because they are highly susceptible to muscle loss. Eating a protein-rich diet and doing strength training with IF is known to speed up the muscle-rebuilding process.

Focus On Getting Enough Electrolytes

Electrolytes like sodium, chloride, potassium, calcium, and magnesium are vital to ensure the normal functioning of our body organs. Since we lose electrolytes through urine and sweat, they need to be replaced quickly. And unlike complete fasting regimens that restrict fluid intake as well, IF allows you to take electrolytes throughout the day.

Electrolyte deficiency can cause nausea, headache, cramps, and irritability during IF. So, lots of electrolyte-rich fluids are recommended.

Consider a Keto Diet Along With IF

Remember, we discussed how IF boosts ketone bodies' production, which serves as a fuel for the brain, heart, and muscles, improves alertness, and lowers inflammation. This is what ketosis is. But that starts about 18 hours into IF. However, incorporating a keto diet in your eating windows can ensure that ketosis begins earlier. This ketosis can improve insulin sensitivity and promote fat loss in menopausal women.

Eat a Nutrient-Dense Diet

To make your small eating windows have a great impact on you, you need to make sure that they are packed with nutrient-rich foods. Incorporation of satiating foods in your eating windows will help you evade hunger during your fasts. To optimize the benefits of IF, you should eat a diet rich in lean proteins, vegetables, and healthy fats.

Celebrity Success Stories

Halle Berry is yet another American actress who is a fan of IF. She revealed her IF plan in November 2018 in a social media post. She revealed that she uses a combination of intermittent fasting and a ketogenic diet to deal with diabetes. These two eating plans help manage her blood sugar levels. Just like Jennifer Aniston, she fasts in the morning and takes her first meal around 2 p.m. She revealed that during her fasting hours, she takes lots of vitamins and minerals to boost her energy levels.

The Lesley Leach Program

The 5:2 fasting method is easy to plan and execute. All you need to do is pick any two days of the week and fast intermittently on those days. Some people fast completely on these days, but the essence of IF suggests you consume a maximum of 500 to 1000 calories on these days.

You can pick any two days between Monday to Sunday for fasting. The rest of the day can be your normal eating days. For instance, if you fast on Friday and Sunday, your planner should look like this:

Week 1						
Monday	Tuesday	Wednesday	Thursday	Friday	Saturday	Sunday
Day 1 with no calorie restriction	Day 2 with no calorie restriction	Day 3 with no calorie restriction	Day 4 with no calorie restrictio n	**Fasting Day 1** Had breakfas t only (500-60 0 cal)	Day 5 with no calorie restriction	**Fasting Day 2** Had a light lunch and a snack (800-100c al)

Given below is a 28-day planner for you to log the details of your 5:2 IF.

Week 1						
Monday	Tuesday	Wednesday	Thursday	Friday	Saturday	Sunday

Week 2						
Monday	Tuesday	Wednesday	Thursday	Friday	Saturday	Sunday

Week 3						
Monday	Tuesday	Wednesday	Thursday	Friday	Saturday	Sunday

Week 4						
Monday	Tuesday	Wednesday	Thursday	Friday	Saturday	Sunday

WILL YOU HELP ME FIGHT BACK?

"To lose confidence in one's body is to lose confidence in oneself."

— SIMONE DE BEAUVOIR

I don't know about you, but I'm tired of all the extreme 'solutions' sold to us by the diet industry. I've seen far too many women in their 50s attempt to boost their health and weight loss, only to come away disheartened.

That's why I wrote this book – and I'd hazard a guess that it's why you're reading it too. Whether you're looking for an alternative to hormone replacement therapy, you've tried diet after diet to no avail, or you're just not sure how to adapt your lifestyle to suit your body's needs at this stage in your life, you're here because you're looking for a solution that really works – one that boosts your confidence rather than chips away at it.

So what I'd like you to do now is help me fight back against the diet industry.

What we have with intermittent fasting is an ancient way of eating that promotes good health and longevity. It has been around for thousands of years... but no one makes any money from it, so the diet industry has nothing to gain from promoting it.

But what we can do is spread the word and promote a healthy lifestyle that's accessible to *everyone*.

By leaving a review of this book on Amazon, you'll help other women discover an alternative and find the guidance they need to succeed with it.

Simply by sharing how this book has helped you and what's contained within it, you'll show other women in their 50s that there's an alternative that really works – and how to find the guidance they need to make a success of it.

Thank you for joining the fight for good health and sustainable weight loss. It truly is much more simple (and effective) than any fad diet would lead us to believe.

Scan the QR code below for a quick review!

5

THE SIDE EFFECTS OF IF AND HOW TO DEAL WITH THEM

IF has gained huge popularity in the last decade, yet it remains a misunderstood diet for many. Opponents of IF reason that it has too many accompanying side effects that outweigh its weight loss benefits, which is why other dieting regimens are far better than IF. However, that's not the case. Most of the side effects of IF are common during the initial days of IF sessions, but once the body gets used to the new routine, they subside on their own. Other side effects develop only when IF is not done properly.

THE DOWNSIDE OF INTERMITTENT FASTING

IF is generally safe for everyone regardless of age and gender, but there are some side effects that newbies can experience. A sudden meal restriction may cause the body to overreact and cause these symptoms. Also, if someone is not properly following the IF protocol, the chances of having these side effects get higher.

Let's have a look at these common side effects of IF.

Hunger Pangs and Cravings

Well! There is no surprise here. Experiencing hunger is the most basic side effect of IF. But that's not something to worry about. A stomach that is used to receiving lots of food throughout the day is bound to show some reactions to sudden changes in the routine. But research has also found that people are more likely to experience hunger during the first few days of fasting in a fasting regimen. Prolonged fasting durations result in a periodic decrease in hunger (Wilhelmi de Toledo et al., 2019). The stomach gradually adjusts to the timing and the number of your meals.

Another issue with IF is that it can create food cravings, and it is problematic because sometimes it can lead some people to develop disordered eating patterns. This effect is more common in people who fail to achieve substantial weight loss through IF. Such people may fast for the required duration but end up eating excessively during the eating windows. Such extreme-level practices can cause rebound weight gain, digestive issues, and malnutrition in some cases.

Digestive Issues

Again, developing digestive issues is a very common side effect of IF. These issues include bloating, nausea, heartburn, constipation, and diarrhea. The sudden routine change that comes with IF is the main cause of these effects.

Boating may be caused because of the changed eating pattern. You see, people often eat speedily during the eating window, which causes them to build gas in their digestive system. Nausea that we may feel during IF may be due to hunger and glucose deficiency. Going too long without food causes a rush of stomach acids, which results in heart-burning sensations. To counter all of these issues, it is best if we break a fast with a light item like a salad or a smoothie. A full meal should be taken one hour after that.

Dehydration is the main cause of several digestive problems during IF. It has been found that people, when restricted from eating, stop consuming fluids too, and this is exactly what happens during the fasting windows. Lack of water in the body causes constipation, headache, and dizziness. Diarrhea may not be the direct result of fasting. It may be because breaking a fast suddenly causes the digestive system to overreact.

Irritability and Mood Changes

Have you ever wondered why we instantly feel good after eating a cookie, candy, or anything sweet? That's because sugar directly triggers our brain to produce the "feel good" hormones that cause us to feel happy and satisfied.

During IF, lowering glucose levels is known to cause irritability, anxiety, and grumpiness. But again, this is something that improves as the body gets used to the long fasting periods. Long fasting hours condition the body to regulate its glucose supply through other non-carbohydrate sources. Watkins & Serpell (2016) reported the same in a study where the participants (52 women) were found to be more irritable during the starting few hours of their 18-hour fast, but by the end of that period, they had achieved a sense of accomplishment and self-control. This corresponds to the positive effects of IF once the body gets used to the IF routine.

Fatigue

It is a general observation that people are tired during fasting hours. That's again because low blood glucose levels lead to an energy deficit. The brain slows down, and the limbs feel drained. Hunger is also known to meddle with normal sleeping patterns, which makes people feel tired during the day.

However, once the body gets used to the fasting routine, these symptoms subside.

Bad Breath

This is one unpleasant side effect of IF, and that is not because of eating habits as most people would think. This is simply because of the lack of saliva production for long periods in IF. Saliva is a natural cleanser that prevents bacterial growth. Another factor that causes bad breath is the ketone body, namely acetone, which is the by-product of fat metabolism. It is known to cause an unpleasant "fruity breath." The rise of acetone in the breath acts as a catalyst for odor-producing bacteria, which eventually leads to bad breath (halitosis).

Drinking lots of water can efficiently deal with this problem by keeping the mouth wet, but since most people forget hydration during IF, this issue occurs often.

Sleep Disturbances

Sleep issues have often been reported with people fasting intermittently, and there are several theories to explain this effect. These issues are more common in the initial fasting days. According to some experts, low glucose levels and associated hunger issues make it hard for people to get a peaceful sleep. Others suggest that excessive loss of electrolytes in urine during the first few days of fasting makes people lethargic and sleepy.

However, one recent study found that fasting does not affect the quality and duration of sleep (Kalam et al., 2021).

Dehydration

This effect is common during the initial days of a fasting session when the body produces excessive urine to deal with the stressed situation created by a lack of glucose in the body. If this fluid is not replaced, severe dehydration can occur.

Dehydration is also common in IF because people forget to consume water during the fasting windows. Dehydration leads to other side effects like headache and nausea. However, this side effect can be easily dealt with by drinking lots of fluids both during fasting and eating windows. Additionally, less consumption of diuretics (things that produce excess urine) can improve water retention in the body.

Headache

Headaches are another common side effect of IF, which resolves on its own once your body has gotten used to the "new system." Headaches experienced during fasting are typically mild and located in the front region of the brain.

Research has revealed that fluctuating blood sugar levels during IF are a common cause of these headaches. Besides, caffeine withdrawal is also reported to be caused during the start of IF sessions (Torelli & Manzoni, 2010).

Malnutrition

This is not something that develops at the beginning of IF. Malnutrition is a condition that develops only when IF is done carelessly without proper protocol. Fasting for extremely long periods and failing to replenish the nutrient reserves could lead to malnutrition. This can also happen when the diet consumed during the eating windows is deficient in the required nutrients.

Malnutrition is not very common in IF because people are generally able to meet their nutrient demands even when the eating hours are limited. Only those who don't plan their meals, eat too little, or follow the same diet for long periods are at risk of malnutrition.

During my IF journey, I have never experienced these side effects for more than three to four days in a row. Taking a healthy diet and maintaining good hydration has always helped my body get over these side effects.

IS INTERMITTENT FASTING LEGIT?

Yes, it is, and you will have a hard time finding a doctor or a nutritionist who suggests otherwise. There is a plethora of research that proves that IF has limitless benefits, and there are thousands of people who are achieving their fitness goals through IF.

The problem with other dieting patterns is that they are hard to stick to, their weight loss effects are temporary, and they do put a lot of food restrictions where you have to count each bite. IF, on the other hand, brings a lot of benefits for both body and mind. It focuses not only on weight loss but also on muscle gain, brain activity, and immunity boosting. And this is done without making you swear off carbs. Besides, it has no strict rules regarding the duration of fasting. You are free to schedule your fast, and you are free to plan your meals.

This is what has made IF the most popular diet among researchers, nutritionists, diet specialists, and people looking for an easy solution to their health issues. IF is especially popular among women because their bodies are not just influenced by their lifestyle choices; hormones play a crucial role too. Such a complicated setup doesn't allow them to follow strict dieting patterns. IF offers a solution by allowing them to balance their hormones and manage their weight without having to endure strict diet controls.

HOW IS INTERMITTENT FASTING DIFFERENT FROM STARVATION?

I think you have got the clarity by now that IF is *not* starvation. This is again something that makes IF the most misunderstood diet pattern of all, and the reason behind that is the strict eating pattern introduced by fad diets. People assume that, like other dieting patterns, IF is also a sophisticated plan that preaches starvation.

IF is not about starvation; it contains no such rules about calorie cutbacks or food restrictions. The idea behind IF is to compel the body to enter the fasting state so that it starts reducing and recycling the unwanted materials that are accumulated over time. IF is not about starving your body; rather, it's about eating meals at certain times during the day and then resting the body to initiate that recycling and healing process. The very definition of IF is sufficient to differentiate it from starvation. According to John Hopkins Medicine (2021), IF is about eating and fasting alternatively. It's about eating and fasting on and off. Research data supports this idea and claims that IF has several benefits regarding metabolic diseases (Moon et al., 2020).

Contrastingly, starvation is about nutrient deprivation. It means going for long periods without food or eating below your body's daily calorie requirements. This calorie deficit may produce weight loss, but that is unsustainable and problematic for the smooth functioning of the body's organs. The notion of starvation has been associated with weight loss because many people are of the view that the quickest way to lose weight is complete nutrient restriction. However, research suggests otherwise. Stark calorie reduction may help in weight loss, especially at the start, but long-term nutrient deficiency initiates a reaction in the body that tries to adapt the system to low energy. This process that follows disturbs not only the weight loss plan but also has detrimental effects on overall health. Let's look at these effects:

- While long-term calorie deprivation may initiate fat metabolism to produce energy (which will cause weight loss), it may also start using muscles as a secondary energy source. This can lead to muscle wasting, which is hard to regain.
- To conserve what little energy stored your body is left with, it starts to lower the rate of metabolism, especially your resting state metabolism (RMR). This means the body is set to consume low calories. While this may be good during the dieting process, the problem arises once the dieting is stopped. So, even when the system is being provided with lots of calories, it is unable to consume most of them. This calorie surplus ultimately leads to rebound weight gain. Therefore, weight maintenance is a lot harder once this restrictive dieting is over. Some recent studies suggest that this low metabolic state ends as soon as the dieting is over, but the accompanying

increased hunger and the elevated urge to eat "freely" causes people to regain weight.

- Another mechanism that your body employs during starvation is making you feel lethargic and dull (Redman & Ravussin, 2011). Opposed to this, no such effects have been reported for IF. It is known to promote alertness and clarity.
- Long-term starvation puts you at a greater risk of developing mental disorders. It is also known to cause psychological eating disorders and binge eating.
- Caloric deficiency affects the immune system as well, making you more susceptible to infections and illnesses.
- Bones start to lose their strength due to the deficiency of required minerals and vitamins.
- In women, menstrual cycles are affected. They are either delayed or stopped completely.
- Other normal functions are slowed down too. For instance, hair and nails become weak, and skin becomes dull.
- Deficiency of vitamins and minerals like vitamins A, D, K, and riboflavin can lead to different disorders that are hard to cure.

I know all of this sounds horrifying, but people still follow these strict dieting in the illusion of quick weight reduction. They may be able to achieve that temporarily, but the effect is not long-lasting. Plus, the side effects of starvation are just too much to deal with. A few of these effects subside as soon as dieting is over, but some of them are hard to reverse.

HOW TO MANAGE HUNGER WHILE FASTING?

We have discussed the potential side effects of fasting, and I know exactly which of these side effects you dread the most. It's hunger and hunger only. You might be thinking, "Okay! I deal with headaches and nausea. I'll take lots of fluids to prevent dehydration. That'll tend to my digestive issues too. But how do I deal with the hunger pangs during the long fasting windows?"

You are right to think that. In fact, most people are reluctant to try IF because they think hunger is too much to deal with. I agree hunger is indeed a part of IF in the beginning, but it is not as bad as you think. If you are committed to this lifestyle and the many benefits it offers, you can and will get through the phase.

Hunger and Intermittent Fasting

First, you need to understand the distinction between appetite and hunger. Our appetite is simply an urge to eat, and it is controlled by several factors, including hormones, senses, and emotions. Conversely, hunger is the *need* to eat, which is often experienced as hunger pangs and stomach grumblings. Second, the hunger experienced during fasting does not get worse with time as most people think. It occurs transiently. You might get hunger pangs for about five to ten minutes at a time. Lastly, feeling hungry during IF is not something you should be worried about. It's completely normal. Sure, you will feel uncomfortable temporarily, but these hunger pangs will subside after a few minutes.

Like other side effects of IF, hunger is also a huge challenge during the first few days because of the appetite that your body is "conditioned" to. But the good part is that this appetite can be reconditioned to tolerate long breaks between meals. The hunger hormone ghrelin is conditioned to release when the brain anticipates meals. This means that the timer in the brain is set to produce ghrelin around meal times only. Of course, this reconditioning takes time, which is why the initial IF is hard. You might get several nudges to eat due to your appetite, and then real hunger will strike in to test your patience. But things will sort out in a few days.

Oh, but wait! There are several tips and tricks that can come in handy when dealing with hunger. These can help you recondition your hunger and assist in maintaining higher energy levels and make you feel satiated for a long time.

Food Hacks

Take a look at the food hacks that might help you deal with hunger during IF.

Eat High-Fat Foods

Eating foods high in healthy fats can promote satiety and help maintain sugar levels for a long time. In fact, the best way to initiate a fast is by eating foods high in protein first, then adding healthy fats next. This promotes the body to rely more on fat rather than carbs to derive energy. Once the body has adapted to fat metabolism, fasting becomes almost effortless. This is one main reason that some IF followers also follow a Ketogenic diet. This will be covered in the next book. 😉

Eat More Protein

We have discussed this before. Proteins also cause satiety because they take a long time to digest. Ingesting a protein-rich meal before starting your fast can make you feel full for a long time.

Limit Alcohol Consumption

Limiting your alcohol consumption, especially on the day before fasting, can help to maintain stable blood sugar levels during fasting. Alcohol is known to cause rapid hormonal changes and fluctuation in blood glucose levels.

Stay Hydrated

Keeping yourself hydrated can help evade hunger. We often confuse thirst with hunger. Often during fasting, when we feel low energy, dry mouth, or parched throat, we think it's probably because we haven't eaten enough. But that's just a sign of low hydration or electrolyte imbalance. Failing to replace the water and electrolytes lost in urine and sweat can cause us to feel "a false hunger." Maintaining higher hydration and electrolyte levels can make our stomach feel "full" and keep our energy levels high.

Take Hot Beverages

Fooling your mind with the "hand to mouth" trick also works very well. For this, I suggest drinking a hot beverage like tea or coffee. Not only will this trick your mind into believing that your stomach is receiving some food, but your stomach will also feel full after getting warmed up by the drink. In fact, it has been proven that decaffeinated coffee reduces hunger by promoting the production of a satiety hormone (Greenberg & Geliebter, 2012). Some people like to add a few drops of coconut oil to their tea. Coconut oil is known to promote ketosis and autophagy. The calories in coconut oil are extremely low and have no impact on insulin levels.

Try Carbonated Water

Carbonated water makes your stomach feel full because of the added carbon dioxide in it.

Try Apple Cider Vinegar (ACV)

ACV is known for its various health benefits. Drinking water with one to two teaspoons of added ACV is known to cause satiety. It is also known to deal with the digestion-related side effects of fasting, like bloating and indigestion.

Life Hacks

Besides using food to solve your hunger issues, there are several other techniques that you can employ to make your fasting windows easier to endure. Several other strategies can help take your mind off food.

Just Avoid Food

Simply smelling food or thinking about it can trigger your cravings. So it is best if you keep away from food during IF. Even seeing food in images can trigger hunger, so it is recommended that during fasting hours, you should *not* be anywhere near food.

Lower Your Stress

Higher stress levels are known to meddle with hormones. This meddling affects the normal production of hunger hormones as well. Therefore, reducing stress can also help you control your hunger.

Sleep Well

Getting good sleep and incorporating some calming exercises in your routine can help lower your stress and control stress-induced hunger.

Keep Yourself Occupied

While appetite may be triggered easily by the smallest of stimuli, masking these cravings is even easier. Simply occupying your brain with a more important task makes it "forget" hunger. Therefore, experts suggest distracting yourself during mealtimes or the last few hours of fasting. This is deemed the easiest trick to deal with hunger. Busying yourself with an activity is also the best way to evade boredom-induced cravings.

Celebrity Success Stories

American socialite Kourtney Kardashian is a huge fan of IF. She expressed her love for IF back in 2018 through a post on her official app where she revealed that she follows an overnight IF plan. For her 16/8 IF, she stops eating at 7 p.m. After fasting for about 15 to 16 hours, she takes her breakfast around 10:30 a.m. to 11 a.m., but only after she is done with her workout session.

She also talked about using a complementary keto diet with IF for a short period, which she discontinued after she noticed some positive changes in her body. Her secret to having hunger-free fasting windows is avocado smoothies and salads packed with fiber.

The Lesley Leach Program

For the 5:2 IF plan, picking two consecutive days is not necessary. You can pick any two days of the week that seem convenient. For instance, if you pick Wednesday and Saturday, your weekly planner should look like this:

Week 1						
Monday	Tuesday	Wednesday	Thursday	Friday	Saturday	Sunday
Day 1 with no calorie restriction	Day 2 with no calorie restriction	**Fasting Day 1** Had breakfast only (500-600 cal)	Day 3 with no calorie restriction	Day 4 with no calorie restriction	**Fasting Day 2** Had a light lunch and Dinner(1 000 cal)	Day 5 with no calorie restrictio n

Given below is a 28-day planner for you to record your 5:2 IF journey.

Week 1						
Monday	Tuesday	Wednesday	Thursday	Friday	Saturday	Sunday

Week 2						
Monday	Tuesday	Wednesday	Thursday	Friday	Saturday	Sunday

Week 3						
Monday	Tuesday	Wednesday	Thursday	Friday	Saturday	Sunday

Week 4						
Monday	Tuesday	Wednesday	Thursday	Friday	Saturday	Sunday

6

TIME TO EAT: SO WHAT SHOULD I EAT?

When I first started IF, the thought that worried me the most was that I had to abandon my favorite foods and stick to a low-salt, no-sugar diet. I thought IF was similar to those fad diets that promise quick results but at the cost of your diet.

Well! IF is nothing like that. It solely focuses on your meal timing. It is based on *when you eat* rather than *what you eat.* The change in body weight brought on by strict dieting is easily achievable through IF without having to make drastic diet changes.

CAN I EAT EVERYTHING I LIKE?

Yes, you can, and that's the best thing about IF. It doesn't implement any kind of restrictions regarding "what to eat?". The calorie deficit that accompanies IF is naturally induced.

Restricting eating to short-eating windows makes sure that you consume fewer calories compared to your normal calorie intake. This reduced calorie count, when combined with other fasting effects, is sufficient to bring about weight loss and other health benefits. So, unless you don't overeat or take a nutrient-poor diet, you can have everything you like.

BEST FOOD COMPONENTS

Let's have a look at some of the most important food components:

Protein

Women over 50 are at high risk of muscle loss. With this muscle loss comes frailty and weakness. Protein is the most important nutrient that can ensure that women maintain a healthy muscle mass. Having a diet rich in proteins can improve the immune system and can help in blood sugar management.

Some protein-rich foods include

- cottage cheese
- buttermilk
- salmon
- lean meat
- plain yogurt
- legumes

- nuts
- seeds

Good Fats

Most people start fearing fats as they age. This shouldn't happen. Fats are not bad for health; it's just the saturated fats you need to avoid. These are the fats that can clog up your blood vessels and cause metabolic disorders. Unsaturated fats pose no such harm. In fact, they are important normal functions of your body. They provide protection to organs, regulate hormonal production, and metabolize some important vitamins. Instead of steering clear of all kinds of fats, you should include a few of these "good" fats in your diet. Rich sources of these fats are

- olive oil
- sesame oil
- avocados and avocado oil
- flaxseeds
- chia seeds
- fish (like Salmon) and other seafood
- grass-fed butter
- nut butter like almond butter
- animal fats (like grass-fed butter, beef tallow, and duck fat)

Low Carbohydrates

Foods with a low percentage of carbohydrates ensure that your body gets the necessary glucose for normal body functioning while encouraging the body to rely more on body fats. They prevent rapid changes in blood glucose levels by releasing glucose solely into the blood. This promotes insulin sensitivity and weight loss and lowers the risk for metabolic diseases. All in all, low glycemic carbs are the best food for your body, especially if you are diabetic or prediabetic. The good thing is there are numerous food sources that are rich in low carbs. These include

- vegetables
- fruits
- whole grains
- milk
- nuts
- legumes
- seeds

Dietary Fiber

Fiber or roughage is technically a form of carbohydrate, but it is categorized separately because it is not digested by the system and passes out as it is. The good part, however, is that it facilitates bowel movements. Eating foods rich in fiber content can relieve constipation and diarrhea, which are quite common during IF.

Rich sources of dietary fiber are

- beans
- lentils
- berries
- apples
- avocado
- broccoli
- whole grains

Vitamins and Minerals

Although vitamins and minerals are required in small amounts, they are extremely important for the smooth functioning of several metabolic processes. Vitamins and minerals are essential to make bones strong, convert food into energy, and regulate fluid movements in and out of the body. Rich sources of vitamins are

- beans\legumes
- dairy products
- fish
- fruits
- vegetables
- grains

Some sources of minerals are

- cereals
- nuts
- fruits
- vegetables
- meat
- dairy products

Probiotics

Probiotics are the sum of beneficial bacteria and fungi that live in your body and fight off the harmful bacteria and neutralize the effects caused by them. You can eat food rich in probiotics to boost your natural bacteria. Excellent sources of probiotics are

- buttermilk
- cheese
- green vegetables
- beans
- legumes
- yogurt
- pickles
- tempeh
- kimchi
- fermented drinks like kombucha

Antioxidants

Oxidative radicals are small molecules that can cause damage to cells and their components and can lead to several types of cancer, cardiac disorders, and premature aging. Antioxidants are the molecules that deal with these oxidative radicals and lower the risk of cellular damage. They are also known to lower cellular inflammation.

Our bodies have their own antioxidants, yet we can also provide them with dietary antioxidants.

Some extra-rich sources of antioxidants are

- herbal teas
- coffee
- chocolate
- fish
- fruits
- Spices and herbs like turmeric, cloves, thyme, rosemary, etc.

HOW TO BREAK A FAST AND BEGIN EATING AGAIN?

You may think that it is the fasting part of your IF routine that is tricky, but it's not; it's how you break the fast that needs you to be cautious because that's the point where the body is highly sensitive to what nutrients you provide it and how. Whatever you eat and the order you eat it in will affect your body's insulin levels and metabolism.

While your daily diet should include all of the nutrients mentioned above, you need to be a little cautious at the time of breaking your fast. I have experimented with a couple of eating patterns before figuring out the exact items that are the best when it comes to breaking a fast. Let's have a look at this pattern:

1. Before you break your fast, you need to lower your fat-burning mode and switch to glucose. To achieve this, you need to lower your cortisol levels (a hormone that promotes fat-burning but also supports fat storage). So before you start eating, you should make sure that it doesn't start storing fats right away. For this, start taking fluid with added salts to lower your cortisol levels. You can take water with Himalayan pink salt or just the normal salt. You can also take bone broth. It will serve the same purpose.
2. To break your fast, take lean proteins. These could be in the form of lean meat, hummus, or any other protein-rich food. Protein shakes are a great option too.
3. Since the metabolism is low due to a long fasting window, you need to boost it as well. For this, I recommend zinc and iodine salts to your food. This will help to lower the risk of hypothyroidism as well.

4. I recommend that you avoid dairy products in the first two hours of your eating window because the calcium and protein in them can cause digestive issues and inflammation. You see, the digestive system is a bit sensitive in the first few hours after fasting. It is also good if you avoid cruciferous vegetables (cabbage, broccoli, brussels sprouts, cabbage, etc.) in the start, too, because the carbs in them can cause bloating.
5. After you have energized your system with proteins, it is good to take carbohydrate-rich food or fat-rich food, but remember not to take both at the same time. Taking them together will cause cells to store fats. Your cells will open for glucose storage, and fats will squeeze in too.
6. Remember, you have to ease your system slowly into working mode. Gobbling up everything will create problems for your metabolic and digestive systems.
7. Two to three hours into your eating window, you can consume anything you want.

BEST FOODS FOR BREAKING A FAST

To prevent nutrient deficiency and to provide proper refueling, nutritionists have recommended a few nutrient-rich foods. Incorporating these in your diet will ensure proper nourishment and make your IF easier. Also, these will optimize the IF benefits for you. It doesn't mean you have to compromise on your comfort foods; just include a couple of these foods in your meals so that you don't miss any of the essential nutrients.

The foods are

- protein-rich
- low-calorie
- low in saturated fats
- low in processed sugars
- high in vitamins, minerals, and antioxidants

Let's have a look at these foods.

Cooked Vegetables

There isn't much difference between cooked and raw vegetables, but research suggests that cooking a few vegetables makes their nutrients easily accessible to the body and preserves the antioxidants in them. Also, steaming or heating them softens them, which makes their digestion easier. Cooked carrots, asparagus, pepper, cabbage, mushrooms, and spinach are a better source of antioxidants when boiled or steamed (Miglio et al., 2008). Besides, vegetables are a great source of vitamins, minerals, and fiber.

Vegetable Juices

Vegetable juices are a quick source of vitamins, minerals, and antioxidants. While there is no scientific evidence that suggests that vegetables are better than whole vegetables, some say that they relieve the body from the fiber-digesting process.

When taken right after breaking a fast, vegetable juice can help in flushing out toxins, lower stress levels, restart the digestive system, and boost the immune system.

Fruits and Smoothies

Raw fruits and fruit smoothies are known to be the best sources of some rare nutrients like folate and several antioxidants. They are rich in minerals, vitamins, and fiber. Raw fruits like apples, bananas, apricots, pears, plums, grapefruit, grapes, and all sorts of berries are known to promote mental health and elevate mood (Brookie et al., 2018). Smoothies made with low-calorie fruits are excellent weight-loss drinks.

Nut Butters

Selection of foods with healthy fats is a difficult task. Most of these good fats are found in conjunction with other nutrients, and the ones that do exist separately are mostly in liquid form. However, nut butter is one such option that provides easy access to healthy fats like omega-3 fatty acids, proteins, antioxidants, and fiber. Cashew butter, peanut butter, and almond butter are some of the most popular options. Adding these to your smoothies, cereals, and snacks can provide a great nutritional punch to your diet.

Fish, Poultry, Meats, and Eggs

All of these are great sources of protein, iron, vitamin B, and zinc, but fish is the most important of them all because it has lean proteins and healthy fats and is easy to digest and metabolize. The rest of the meats may not be fat-free, but you can choose lean meats like bottom round or top round of beef and pork to avoid these fats. You can trim fat from meat and skin the chicken to remove unhealthy fat attached to it.

Egg whites are a great source of protein and iron. Adding them to your meals can help meet your daily protein requirement.

Bone Broth and Soups

Bone broths and soup are options for starting your eating window. They are low in calories but rich in minerals, vitamins, electrolytes, and proteins, but bone broth has added nutrients like collagen and chondroitin, which can help lower inflammation and strengthen bones.

Leafy Greens

Leafy green vegetables are rich in all beneficial nutrients, including vitamins, minerals, antioxidants, and fiber. Eating these vegetables two to three hours into your eating window ensures that your body recovers its energy reserves and gets enough fiber to facilitate smooth bowel movements.

Arugula, watercress, cabbage, spinach, collard greens, and kale are some leafy greens that you can incorporate into your diet.

Fermented Foods

Simple fermented foods like pickles, sauerkraut, kimchi, and kefir can help boost your good bacteria, provide a boost to your immune system, and improve digestion. These foods need no time for preparation and can be stored for a long time.

Celebrity Success Stories

IF is not some low-yielding method that takes a lot of time and effort to bear results. It starts showing tangible effects in a matter of weeks, and this is evident from the IF routine of the actress Scarlett Johansson who used a combination of IF and strength training to meet the requirements for her fast and fit character Black Widow in The Avengers movie series.

Her fasting windows started from 9 p.m. and stretched for 12 hours, but sometimes they were pushed beyond that due to the filming schedule. On such days, she fasted for 14 to 15 hours straight.

The Lesley Leach Program

The 14:10 method of IF is one of the smoothest and easiest to follow, especially when most of the fasting window is spent while sleeping. This method is also suitable for those suffering from metabolic disorders like type 2 diabetes.

Planning the 14:10 IF regimen is easy. All you have to do is to decide when you want to begin your 10-hour eating window. The rest of the period is your fasting period. For instance, if you pick an eating window between 9 a.m. to 7 p.m., your schedule might look like this:

1. 9 a.m. Breakfast
2. 1 p.m. Lunch
3. 4 p.m. Snack Time
4. 6:30 p.m. Dinner

Your weekly 14:10 IF schedule might look like this:

14:10 Plan	**Day 1**	**Day 2**	**Day 3**	**Day 4**	**Day 5**	**Day 6**	**Day 7**
6 a.m.	**Fasting**	**Fasting**	**Fasting**	**Fasting**	**Fasting**	**Fasting**	**Fasting**
7 a.m.	**window**	**window**	**window**	**window**	**window**	**window**	**window**
8 a.m.							
9 a.m.	Breakfast	Breakfast	Breakfast	Breakfast	Breakfast	Breakfast	Breakfast
10 a.m.							
11 a.m.							
Noon.							
1 p.m.	Lunch	Lunch	Lunch	Lunch	Lunch	Lunch	Lunch
2 p.m.							
3 p.m.							
4 p.m.	Snack	Snack	Snack	Snack	Snack	Snack	Snack
5 p.m.							
6 p.m.	Dinner	Dinner	Dinner	Dinner	Dinner	Dinner	Dinner
7 p.m.	**Fasting**	**Fasting**	**Fasting**	**Fasting**	**Fasting**	**Fasting**	**Fasting**
8 p.m.	**window**	**window**	**window**	**window**	**window**	**window**	**window**
9 p.m.	**begins**	**begins**	**begins**	**begins**	**begins**	**begins**	**begins**
10 p.m.	.	.	.	.	.	.	.
11 p.m.	.	.	.	.	.	.	.
Midnig	.	.	.	.	.	.	.
ht	.	.	.	.	.	.	.
1 a.m.	.	.	.	.	.	.	.
2 a.m.	.	.	.	.	.	.	.
3 a.m.	.	.	.	.	.	.	.
4 a.m.	.	.	.	.	.	.	.
5 a.m.							

You can use the 14:10 IF planner below to schedule your eating and fasting windows as well as to plan your meals during the eating hours.

14:10 Plan	Day 1	Day 2	Day 3	Day 4	Day 5	Day 6	Day 7
6 a.m. 7 a.m. 8 a.m. 9 a.m. 10 a.m. 11 a.m. Noon. 1 p.m. 2 p.m. 3 p.m. 4 p.m. 5 p.m. 6 p.m. 7 p.m. 8 p.m. 9 p.m. 10 p.m. 11 p.m. Midnig ht 1 a.m. 2 a.m. 3 a.m. 4 a.m. 5 a.m.							

14:10 Plan	**Day 8**	**Day 9**	**Day 10**	**Day 11**	**Day 12**	**Day 13**	**Day 14**
6 a.m. 7 a.m. 8 a.m. 9 a.m. 10 a.m. 11 a.m. Noon. 1 p.m. 2 p.m. 3 p.m. 4 p.m. 5 p.m. 6 p.m. 7 p.m. 8 p.m. 9 p.m. 10 p.m. 11 p.m. Midnig ht 1 a.m. 2 a.m. 3 a.m. 4 a.m. 5 a.m.							

14:10 Plan	**Day 15**	**Day 16**	**Day 17**	**Day 18**	**Day 19**	**Day 20**	**Day 21**
6 a.m. 7 a.m. 8 a.m. 9 a.m. 10 a.m. 11 a.m. Noon. 1 p.m. 2 p.m. 3 p.m. 4 p.m. 5 p.m. 6 p.m. 7 p.m. 8 p.m. 9 p.m. 10 p.m. 11 p.m. Midnig ht 1 a.m. 2 a.m. 3 a.m. 4 a.m. 5 a.m.							

14:10 Plan	Day 22	Day 23	Day 24	Day 25	Day 26	Day 27	Day 28
6 a.m. 7 a.m. 8 a.m. 9 a.m. 10 a.m. 11 a.m. Noon. 1 p.m. 2 p.m. 3 p.m. 4 p.m. 5 p.m. 6 p.m. 7 p.m. 8 p.m. 9 p.m. 10 p.m. 11 p.m. Midnig ht 1 a.m. 2 a.m. 3 a.m. 4 a.m. 5 a.m.							

7

FASTING MADE EASY: DON'T OVERTHINK IT JUST DO IT!

There are a variety of weight loss methods out there with varying levels of efficacy, but when it comes to women over 50, there are certain factors that create hindrances. The most important of these factors is slow metabolism which stems from decreased lean muscle mass. This leads to a less active lifestyle, and that's when body fat starts accumulating.

Intermittent fasting is the best plan in this regard because it is not just a plan that targets calories; it offers a range of health benefits, all of which act synergistically to ensure that metabolism is improved, mental health is enhanced, and the risk of several age-related disorders is lowered.

5 TIPS TO START IF

Intermittent fasting is a lot easier said than done. The excess of information related to IF methods, meal plans, and related lifestyle changes make this process even more confusing. Now that you have got the details about several IF variants and recommended foods let's look at an easy five-step plan that will help you ace your IF journey.

Identify Personal Goals

You must not start IF just because "everybody" is doing it. The reason for choosing IF should be a personal one. To ensure success with IF, there should be a solid reason behind it. People choose IF for several reasons; some do it because they want to lose weight, and others to build muscle. Some opt for IF to lower the risk of a certain metabolic disease. Women often use it to balance their hormones. So before you start deciding other details regarding your IF plan, sit down and answer these questions:

1. Why do you want to fast intermittently?
2. What do you want to achieve through IF?
3. Are there any personal goals that you want to achieve through it, or do you want to impress others?

Setting a few goals before initiating IF will motivate you throughout the process and give you the strength to withstand the hard phases of this process.

Figure Out Your IF Plan

This is the most crucial step. Figuring out the best plan for yourself will streamline the rest of the process for you. This will allow your body to adapt easily to the changes, and you will face minimal side effects.

The question is, how do you know which one is the best IF method for you?

For this, I recommend starting with an easy method. Instead of jumping straight to the 16/8 variant, start with a smaller fasting window, like a 10 to 12 hours window, and gradually increase its duration. Stick to an IF variant for at least a month to see how your body is responding to it.

For people suffering from a metabolic disorder, it is better if they consult with a doctor before switching to an extreme fasting method.

Figure Out Your Calorie Needs

Even when there are no inherent calorie restrictions in IF, there needs to be a calorie deficit during the whole fasting regimen that can promote the weight loss effects of IF. Regarding that, there are no strict diet plans. However, you need to make sure that whatever you are eating is contributing to a net calorie deficit. Generally, the fasting schedule is sufficient to create this deficit. The short eating window ensures that you are eating less than you normally do. Additionally, you can opt for foods that are nutrient-rich but low in calories to help you tolerate long fasting hours while promoting fat-burning. Simply drinking a glass of water before your meals will make you feel full and result in less calorie consumption. Reducing the size of the portions of your meals (especially those rich in carbs) will also help in creating an overall calorie deficit.

Figure Out Your Meal Plan

Again, there are no specific requirements regarding meal planning in IF, but meal planning ahead of initiating a fasting program will allow you to incorporate more nutritious meals into your diet. This will allow you to make conscious decisions about your diet.

It is all right if you prefer spontaneous eating in your eating windows, but a conscious effort to plan your meals will allow you to keep a check on your calorie intake. Carefully deciding what to put on your plate will save you a few bucks since you will be wasting less food.

Optimize the Effects of IF

The flexibility of the IF schedule is what makes it fun. This flexibility allows you to incorporate some changes in your IF routine, and these changes could serve to optimize the benefits and efficacy of IF for you. You can include a workout routine in your IF regimen. This will help you gain muscle mass, provide flexibility in your joints, and speed-up fat metabolism. Adding high-volume but low-calorie foods to your diet will allow you to fast comfortably for longer durations. Maintaining high hydration levels will flush out toxins from the body, provide you with plump skin and help you deal with hunger pangs during IF.

PAY ATTENTION TO YOUR BODY

Hormonal changes in women are known to lower their muscle mass and body strength. This sufficiently weakens their joints and makes their movement restricted.

To deal effectively with age-related issues, bringing changes in lifestyle, diet, and physical activity is important. While IF effectively deals with the first two changes, the incorporation of a workout routine is necessary to ensure that you do sufficient physical activity during your day.

IF targets your hormones, blood glucose levels, and vital organs to bring about all the beneficial changes in your body but complementing this IF with a workout routine is known to optimize these benefits and help you gain lean muscle mass. While experts support exercising with IF, they are of the view that it should be done safely and effectively.

Can You Exercise While Fasting?

This is an important query to address before you start your IF journey. Many women are already following a workout routine and others want to do so once they start fasting. And the answer is simply yes! You can exercise while fasting. But it depends on how you feel and how your body responds to it.

There are a few issues regarding exercising that need serious consideration to ensure safety and effectiveness.

Benefits and Risks of Exercising During IF

The evidence regarding the benefits of exercising is very encouraging. However, exercising during fasting intermittently involves certain risks. Let's get to the benefits first.

As far as weight loss is concerned, working out on an empty stomach is known to cause rapid fat-burning. The same logic applies to working out in a fasted state. Physical activity during exercise causes an early depletion of glycogen stores, and so the body is forced to rely on fat metabolism rather than carbohydrates. (Bachman et al., 2016).

However, there is an ongoing debate on the best time to work out during fasting. Some say that physical exertion at the start of the fasting window causes an early depletion of energy stores and slows down metabolism. They suggest working out in the last few hours of IF.

The other group of experts proposes that since weight loss and detoxification are the primary goals of IF, working out right after eating will help initiate fat oxidation and autophagy sooner in the fasting window.

Research has also revealed that exercise training is one of the best intervention methods that can help women regain the muscle mass lost during menopause and prevent loss of muscle function with advancing age. Both IF and strength training act synergistically to rebuild muscle fibers. Strength training creates micro-tears in wasted muscle fibers, and IF redirects dietary proteins to these micro-tears, where they rebuild these muscles to be stronger and larger. The combined effect of IF and exercising is also known to lower early signs of aging and slow down disease progression (Anton et al., 2018).

Besides these benefits, there are some risks too. In the absence of proper nutrition, exercising can initiate muscle breakdown and use the resulting proteins as fuel. Overexertion during workout sessions can also lead to a quick energy drain and make you feel lethargic for the rest of your fasting period.

Considering everything, it's best if you decide the intensity and duration of your workout session based on your body's response. You will need to employ a trial-and-error method for that. Try a combination of workouts to decide what works best for you.

What Is the Best Time to Workout?

This is a relative subject. There is no recommended best time for working out along with IF. Research reveals that there is no clear difference in body composition between people who work out during the fasting window and those who work out after breaking their fast (Schoenfeld et al., 2014). Most people like to work out right after eating to speed up fat metabolism but also because they can perform well with high energy. Others do it right before breaking their fast. This allows them to regain their strength right after the workout sessions.

However, in the case of patients suffering from metabolic disease, working out right after eating is recommended.

Make Your Workout Sessions Safe and Effective

While combining workout sessions with IF, your fitness and ease should be your priority. It would be best if you opted for a method that's easy to sustain. You need to stay in the safe zone. Here are a few tips to help you with that.

Workout Close to Your Meal Timings

That's the golden rule for all workout sessions. Your body should have access to high energy during the workout session or should be refueled soon after the workout session. Eating right after working out will provide your body regain its strength and aid in muscle regeneration. On the other hand, working out right after meals will ensure an energetic performance during the whole session. This is even more important if you are in strength training.

Maintain a High Hydration and Electrolyte Level

Due to excessive sweating and rapid fat-burning, there is a constant energy drain during strength training. This makes you feel hunger and thirst immediately after workout sessions. Excessive loss of electrolytes through sweating makes you feel lethargic and dull. To deal with all of these issues, maintaining a higher hydration level is your only option. Adding electrolytes to your drinks can help you deal with lightheadedness and lethargy.

Opt for the Easiest Workout Combination

Pushing yourself too hard won't speed up the weight loss or muscle-building process; it will simply cause you to burn out. You feel dizzy, hungry, and exhausted during IF. Instead, opting for an easy workout routine will create positive effects on your body and mind.

Pick a Workout Routine Based on Your IF Method and Your Diet

Use your IF method as a guide to select a workout session for you. If your IF routine has a short eating window like the warrior diet, opt for a low-intensity workout. For example, walking daily or at least three times a week for 30min. Even yoga or riding a bike are great ways to start. It's really all about moving your body. If you are doing 16/8 IF, you can opt for a more intense strength training routine.

The type of nutrients that you have in your diet can also act as a guide for a workout type. Strength workouts generally require more energy and therefore, the days you have a high-carb diet are the best to do strength training. However, HIIT and Cardio can be done with a low-carb diet. Again, we all will have different results, so find what works for you and which fasting schedule gets you the results you seek.

Listen to Your Body

This is the best way to gauge your progress when exercising with IF. If your body responds negatively to workout sessions by making you feel dizzy, weak, or nauseated, this means you need to STOP. Next, rethink your nutrition and, most importantly, your hydration status. Low electrolytes could be the culprit here. As soon as you feel ready, you can start again, but with an easy workout session.

Remember, the aim of your workout sessions is to optimize the effects of IF, not to lower them. For some women, exercising will work perfectly with IF; for others, not so well, at least in the beginning. But even if that's the case, women don't give up. Try less intense workouts like beginner yoga, stretching, and even swimming to work your muscles and joints.

As far as your exercise options are concerned, there are many, and each one has benefits of its own. Let's look at them.

HIIT

Merriam-Webster defines HIIT as "a form of training that alternates between periods of intense exercise with periods of less intense exercise." The period of intense exercise lasts for 20 to 40 seconds, while the less intense exercise period lasts for 15 to 30 seconds. A HIIT session may look like this:

1. Squatting for 20 seconds.
2. Running at full speed for 20 seconds.
3. Static (standing in one place) jogging for 20 seconds.
4. Forward-stepping lunges for 40 seconds (alternating legs after 20 seconds).
5. Sprinting on a stationary bicycle for 20 seconds.
6. Jumping jacks for 20 seconds.

Or simply, one exercise or activity can be repeated several times with alternating speeds.

The alternating durations of intense training with low-intensity exercises create a rapid rise in metabolism. The impact of this workout is similar to intense training sessions. HIIT is a good option for those who find it hard to spare time for exercise in their daily routine. Plus, it entails no specific workout step. You can combine a variety of exercises and activities to build a regimen of your own.

Let's see how HIIT helps us achieve our fitness and health goals.

One of the biggest pros of HIIT is its efficiency. It burns 25-30% more calories than other forms of exercise but with 30% less effort (Falcone et al., 2015).

HIIT promotes the fat-burning process steadily. These effects are not limited to the workout session; HIIT continues to increase metabolic rate hours after the workout session is done. This is one of the reasons why HIIT is recommended in the first few hours of the fasting window. It burns calories faster and initiates a fat-burning process that continues for the rest of the fasting period. According to Abbasi et al. (2020), both IF and HIIT improve lipid profiles, and having a low lipid profile is directly related to lowered diabetes, Cardiovascular diseases (CVD), and cancer risk.

HIIT offers an easy solution for obese and overweight individuals who want to lose fat with relatively shorter workout sessions. Women looking for easy ways to reduce their waist circumference can benefit from HIIT.

The effect of HIIT on muscle health is monumental. It helps strengthen the muscles that are worked efficiently during the workout session. These involve the leg and trunk muscles. A rather surprising study shows that formerly inactive individuals stand to gain more muscle mass from HIIT than those who are already living an active lifestyle (Damas et al., 2015). So if you are a woman who is new to IF or exercising, you have a greater chance of gaining lean muscle mass through HIIT. The ability of muscles to consume oxygen has a direct impact on their health. HIIT is known to improve this oxygen consumption capacity too. Normally, this requires continuous intense activity, but with HIIT, the same results are produced within a short time.

Lastly, HIIT is a great option for individuals suffering from metabolic diseases, especially those who are obese and have mobility issues. Engaging in a combination of easy-to-do exercises can help you burn body fat, lower blood pressure, and manage blood glucose levels.

CARDIO

Cardio is short for Cardiovascular exercises, and the idea behind these is to target the heart to beat faster, which in turn boosts metabolism and burns calories. Cardio serves the dual function of burning fat and building lean muscle mass. You start by working your core muscles, which then demand more oxygen and energy to sustain the process. This results in increased breathing rate and heart rate. There are several exercises that you can do as part of your cardio sessions, including

- jogging
- running
- cycling
- bear crawling
- dancing
- rowing
- canoeing
- swimming
- body squats
- jumping rope
- skating (including roller skating, ice skating, and inline skating)
- hiking, etc.

Doing cardio in the fasted state is a great way to burn body fat without causing any damage to muscles. The complete absence of carb-based fuel during the last few hours of IF compels the system to rely on fat reserve, which boosts the fat oxidation process. I prefer cardio in the mornings because 8-12 hours of sleep pushes the body into a fasted state, making it a perfect target for cardio exercises.

However, if building new muscle mass is your goal, I suggest eating before a cardio session. Working out on an empty stomach is okay if you are trying to lose body fat. Lack of energy during cardio will shift the body towards fat metabolism without harming muscle mass; proteins are not a desirable energy source. But when you want to gain lean muscle mass, working out after a protein-rich meal will stimulate muscle fiber construction. However, if you have a slow digestive system, I suggest you perform cardio on an empty stomach since working with a full stomach may make you feel sick.

For the best result, I suggest opting for low to medium-intensity cardio workouts. Also, to avoid dehydration and related health issues, you should drink plenty of water before and after the workout sessions.

STRENGTH TRAINING

According to Merriam-Webster, strength training includes activities that build muscles. The idea behind strength training is to make the muscles do extra work against resistance (provided by heavy weights and stretching). Continuous subjection to this resistance increases their endurance and strength. This resistance can be provided through several techniques, including free weights, weight machines, resistance bands, suspension equipment, and one's own body weight.

The most important benefit of strength training is improved muscle mass and strength. It gradually builds flexibility in major joints by increasing their range of rotation, flexion, and extension. This is something that gets hard with advancing age, and maintaining these abilities can lower the risk of injury and immobility. Strength training creates an elaborate weight-management setup that not only burns fat but also causes muscle gain. As you build more muscles, you burn more fat, even at rest. This fat-burning reduces the risk of mental and metabolic disorders. Strength training is also known to have positive cognitive and mental effects too. It lowers the risk of mental decline, depression, and memory loss and creates a positive self-image.

All of the above-mentioned benefits of strength training are easily achievable even when done in conjunction with IF. However, muscle gain is a tricky subject that requires effective oversight. The underlying mechanism that repairs micro-tears in muscles and rebuilds muscle fibers requires high dietary proteins to work effectively. In the absence of these proteins, strength training will only cause muscle deterioration. Therefore, the ideal time to do strength training is during the eating window or right before breaking a fast so that dietary proteins (and carbohydrates) are available to assist the recovery process. Trying a strength training session, for the first time, on an empty stomach may cause lethargy and compromises workout performance.

To do strength training safely and effectively, keeping the workout sessions short is always a good idea. To decrease the duration of a session, you can simply reduce the number of reps for each exercise. Paying attention to body response is the best way to gauge the safety levels of strength training.

You should always stop if you feel like an exercise is straining the muscles or making you feel dizzy all of a sudden. Lastly, maintaining high levels of hydration will help you get through the workout sessions.

MEAL SCHEDULING FOR INTERMITTENT FASTING

We have discussed in detail how the fasting windows work, what you can do during fasting windows to reap the maximum benefits of fasting, and how you can pass this time without stressing your body. But what about the eating windows? Sure, the idea of eating windows seems fun. It seems easy. All you have to do is eat your fill. But most of the IF newbies find the idea of meal planning a bit overwhelming.

However, meal planning for IF is a lot easier than dieting plans, where strict calorie restriction is required. Once you start IF, you will feel that effective meal planning can make you feel fuller during the fasting hours and make your meals as simple as possible.

I have broken down fasting schedules and meal plans into several tiers, from beginner level to level pro. Following these will help you ease into IF meal planning.

Beginner Level

For IF newbies, I recommend a modified form of the 16/8 method, which includes a 10-hour eating window and a 14-hour fast making it 14/10. Interestingly, this modified form allows you to fit all three of your meals plus a snack in a 10-hour eating window.

To start an eating window, I recommend a cup of soup or bone broth. Take something that is easy on your stomach. I prefer having a peanut butter protein smoothie, and sometimes I top it with some healthy fats like coconut oil or avocado oil.

With a gap of three to four hours, you can have your second meal of the day. For this meal, you have a variety of options. You can also eat your favorite foods at this point in your eating window. My preferred options are grass-fed beef burgers, vegetable salad topped with white meat chunks, and lentil and vegetable soup. I like to have green tea right after that.

For snack time, I prefer dark chocolate-covered almonds. This helps curb my sweet tooth, plus the sugar and fat in them sustain me till dinner.

Lastly, for my dinner, I like to fill up on foods that keep me satiated for a long time. Salmon air-fried in avocado oil or a juicy Ribeye steak is my favorite dinner option. Besides that, I like having soup or a dinner salad.

Intermediate Level

Starting with a 14/10 IF, you can slowly increase the duration of your eating window to 16 hours. A 16/8 IF will allow you to have two meals and a snack in your eating window. For your first meal, you can have a small meal that is rich in proteins and carbs. With a gap of three hours, you can have a snack. Lastly, you can have your dinner rich in proteins, fiber, and fats.

Intermediate-level IF is easy to do, and once your body has adapted well to this kind of fasting routine, you can switch to more intense fasting regimens. For starters, you can switch to the 18/6 IF plan.

Advanced Level

For an advanced level of fasting, you can have a 5:2 meal plan that entails a calorie restriction of up to 500-700 calories on two days of the week. For the rest of the week, you can follow your normal calorie intake. Since 1800-2200 calories are the normal requirement for women over 50 (Skolnik & King, 2005), one way to restrict these to 500-700 calories is by reducing your meals by 1/3rd.

During the fasting days, you can have two small meals or a large meal along with a snack.

Super Advanced Level

For the super-advanced level, you can try IF variants that involve only one meal a day. These include the warrior diet and OMAD. These IF methods will require you to plan one single nutrient-rich meal. To meet your nutritional requirements, you will require a meal plan that incorporates all of the basic nutrients in one meal.

Pro Level

This is the ultimate level of IF. I recommend alternate-day fasting (ADF) and extended fasting for pro-level IF. To be able to fast for 24-48 hours, you will require stamina and strength to withstand hunger. Meals after such a long duration should be rich in carbs, protein, fats, and essential vitamins and minerals.

WEEKLY IF MEAL PLANNER

IF is not about using calorie calculators to keep track of how much you are eating, but when it comes to keeping track of time, IF has rules. In fact, the whole idea of improving metabolism and promoting fat oxidation during IF is based on time-restricted eating. If you have set particular timings for your eating windows, you need to finish your meals within that window. Following strict timings during IF helps the body adapt to metabolic changes and tolerate hunger.

For instance, if you have set your eating window from 8 a.m. to 2 p.m., you shouldn't break your fast at 7:30 a.m. and shouldn't be eating past 2 p.m. A little relaxation in the first few days is okay, but in the long run, you should adhere to the schedule.

To keep track of my fasting schedule during the day, I use a simple planner where I log my fasting and eating hours and the number of meals that I have each day. To ensure that I am eating a diverse diet, I like to jot down what I eat every day. This weekly meal planner helps me to remember the groceries that I need for my meal preparations. Have a look at my weekly 18/6 IF meal planner. During this plan, I like to have a smoothie (for my breakfast), a snack, and a complete lunch.

Weekly Meal Planner					
18/6 IF Meal Planner	**Breakfast (8-8:30 a.m.)**	**Snack (10-11 a.m.)**	**Lunch (1-2 p.m.)**	**Snack**	**Dinner**
Monday	Strawberry and mint smoothie	Apple with pistachios	Lentil soup, Chicken curry with rice		
Tuesday	Green vegetable smoothie	Nuts and raisins	Grass-fed beef burgers		
Wednesday	Kale smoothie with chia seeds	Banana with peanut butter	Green vegetable salad, Grilled chicken breasts		
Thursday	Peach and Mint Smoothie	Granola bar	Tomato soup, Vegetable sandwich		
Friday	Blueberries Smoothie	Kale chips	Baked potatoes stuffed with chicken and cheese		
Saturday	Green Vegetables Smoothie	Greek yogurt	Lentil curry with rice, smoked Salmon		
Sunday	Banana and Berries Smoothie	Strawberries and chocolate chip cookies	Baked red beans, Chicken fried steaks		

You can use the same planner to plan your meals for IF.

Weekly Meal Planner					
IF method ( )	**Breakfast ( )**	**Snack ( )**	**Lunch ( )**	**Snack ( )**	**Dinner ( )**
Monday					
Tuesday					
Wednesday					
Thursday					
Friday					
Saturday					
Sunday					

Celebrity Success Stories

American actress and producer Reese Witherspoon rely on low-calorie drinks like coffee and "green juice" to limit her calories in the mornings. Following in the footsteps of her

Friends co-star, Jennifer Aniston, she fasts for almost 16 hours daily for six days a week. She likes to wake up at 5:30 in the morning and works out with her kids. She likes to have at least one cheat day a week.

The Lesley Leach Program

Planning an alternate-day fasting (ADF) schedule is easy. All you have to do is eat normally on one day and fast on the next. Something like this:

- Day 1-Eat normally.
- Day 2-Fast intermittently (consume 500-600 calories).
- Day 3-Eat normally.
- Day 4-Fast intermittently (consume 500-600 calories).
- And repeat.

Given below is a 28-day ADF planner for you to keep track of your fasting progress and log your daily caloric intake.

My ADF plan	Day 1	Day 2	Day 3	Day 4	Day 5	Day 6	Day 7
Normal day or Fasting day							
F o o d s consumed througho ut the day							

My ADF plan	Day 8	Day 9	Day 10	Day 11	Day 12	Day 13	Day 14
Normal day or Fasting day							
F o o d s consumed througho ut the day							

My ADF plan	Day 15	Day 16	Day 17	Day 18	Day 19	Day 20	Day 21
Normal day or Fasting day							
Foods consumed throughout the day							

My ADF plan	Day 22	Day 23	Day 24	Day 25	Day 26	Day 27	Day 28
Normal day or Fasting day							
Foods consumed throughout the day							

8

IF MISTAKES AND HOW TO AVOID THEM

After going through the contents of this book, you should be well-equipped with all the basics of IF and ready to start your own IF journey. But before you do that, I want to share some common mistakes that most newbies commit. However small, these mistakes can not only sabotage your weight loss efforts but can severely damage your overall health.

Keep the following points in mind to ensure that you are doing everything in a proper way to reap the benefits of IF.

STARTING DRASTICALLY WITH IF

This is the most common mistake that people make. Our bodies are not very quick when it comes to adapting to drastic changes. Just like overeating throws our digestive system out of balance, suddenly switching from five meals to two meals will result in severe side effects. In extreme cases, the body enters starvation mode, and that's when it starts breaking down muscles instead of strengthening them. Surely, we don't want that.

So, instead of jumping right to an intense form of IF, I suggest you start by gradually increasing the interval between your meals. This will help you determine how long you can go without eating. Once you have done so, you can try to reduce the number of your daily meals before actually trying an IF plan. This strategy will help you lower the IF-related side effects.

CHOOSING THE WRONG FASTING PLAN

One of the misconceptions regarding the selection of IF plans is that they are thought to be the same, and therefore when it comes to the selection of an IF plan, people don't pay much attention to how it will affect their normal routine. The wrong selection of an IF plan can severely affect your adherence to the plan and lower the benefits of IF as a whole. For instance, if you are a foodie, a sudden jump to a 20/4 plan will severely affect your energy levels, and you may have to face side effects like dizziness, nausea, and irritability. Likewise, if you are a night owl, starting your fasting windows in the evenings is not a good idea and if you are extremely busy in the office from 8 a.m. to 2 p.m., scheduling an eating window between these hours is not a viable option.

To avoid these issues, you need to select a plan that fits your daily routine without affecting your working hours and sleep-wake cycle. Select an IF plan that offers you the flexibility to enjoy meals with your family and friends.

OVEREATING RIGHT AFTER YOU BREAK A FAST

Feeling the urge to reward your fasting efforts during the eating window is very common, especially for those who are new to IF. This mistake leads people to do overeating which not only causes a sudden rise in insulin levels but also ruins the aim of IF. Burdening the digestive system after such a long resting phase causes it to overreact, and this leads to problems like bloating acidity, diarrhea, constipation, and nausea.

To avoid these issues, you need to replenish your energy stores periodically. Instead of starting your eating window with high-carbs and fat-rich food, you should stick to light smoothies and salads. Even when there are no strict calorie restrictions in IF, yet you should make sure that you normally eat during the eating window and *not overeat.* Chewing food well and drinking lots of water can help lower gut-related side effects.

EATING TOO LITTLE BEFORE THE FASTING WINDOW

To ensure hunger-free fasting windows, you need to eat well during the last few hours of your eating windows. In a bid to lower their total calorie intake, people often end up eating too little during their eating hours. Not eating sufficiently can result in an early release of hunger hormones which can make you miserable for the rest of your fasting hours. In the long run, this condition can lead the body to enter starvation mode, which can be a major setback for your weight loss plan.

Taking a meal rich in proteins, healthy fats, vitamins, minerals, and fiber can help you steer clear of such a situation.

UNKNOWINGLY BREAKING THE INTERMITTENT FAST

IF newbies should keep track of drinks and supplements that break a fast because several such items may seem calorie-free but are not. The Rule of thumb is anything with calories can break your fast. However, even the professionals say 30-50 calories is ok. Let's look at a list of these items that you need to steer clear of during fasting windows:

- fruit juice concentrate
- pectin and maltodextrin-containing drinks
- protein powders

- protein-containing energy drinks
- multivitamins containing sugars or extra fillers
- drinks containing high-calorie fats (coconut oil is okay!)

Taking any item that contains added calories and digestible carbs can jerk your body out of the fasting state, cause insulin levels to spike, and halt autophagy. Therefore, it's necessary to make sure that you are consuming calorie-free drinks and supplements during your fasting windows.

CHOOSING UNHEALTHY FOOD DURING YOUR FEASTING WINDOW

Just like eating too little can cause problems for you. Similarly, consuming unhealthy foods can create problems for your fasting body. After going for a long period without meals, your body needs all the goodies to decrease its energy deficit and to refuel itself for the next session of fasting. However, when you opt for foods containing processed carbs and saturated fats, you not only sabotage your fasting efforts but also create a negative impact on your metabolism. Such foods shift the metabolism towards carbohydrates. The resulting rush in insulin may make you feel full for a short period, but soon after that hunger hormone will kick in and make you hungry too soon into the fasting window.

To avoid this issue, your last meals of the day should be rich in complex carbohydrates, healthy fats, lean proteins, and fiber content.

NOT DRINKING ENOUGH WATER

When you are off calories, hydration is your best buddy that can get you through your fasting windows without feeling energy deficit, hunger, and lethargy. Our water requirements are not only met with the water we drink; some of this water comes from the food we consume. So, when we are consuming any food, we have to make up for that water loss through extra consumption of water. It is, therefore, highly recommended that you drink more water on fasting days than you normally do.

Also, too much consumption of caffeinated drinks causes more urine production, which then causes more water loss. To prevent this, caffeinated drinks should be consumed in a controlled amount.

MAKING POOR LIFESTYLE CHOICES

IF is not simply a diet plan; rather, it is a lifestyle that involves adopting a number of healthy habits and abandoning the bad ones. IF not just targets your eating pattern, it provides you with several other opportunities to rest your body and cleanse it of unwanted accumulations. Unhealthy lifestyle habits like not getting enough sleep, junk food binging, smoking, drinking, and being inactive can negatively impact the results of IF.

Therefore, it is advised that besides IF, you should try to change your unhealthy habits so as to maximize IF benefits.

NOT EXERCISING

IF is not like a hunger strike where people just sit and avoid eating anything. In the case of IF, staying inactive will negatively affect the IF outcomes. While the idea of IF is to promote weight loss and muscle building, staying inactive will push the body to store more fat and push the body to consume muscle proteins in case of starvation.

To make sure that your body is responding positively to IF, make sure that you incorporate a workout routine in your IF plan.

GIVING UP TOO SOON

IF is not like a magic bean that'll grow overnight. It takes time to reap its effects, but people get easily discouraged by the slow progress and abandon the plan. Losing stubborn fat takes even more time in the 50s when the metabolism gets slower, and the activity rate is low.

You may lose weight rapidly in the first few weeks of IF; after that, the process will slow down. You will need patience and strict adherence to see some tangible changes in your body. You will make several mistakes along the way, but learning from those mistakes and embracing changes in your body along every step will help you get better at IF.

Celebrity Success Stories

Vanessa Hudgens revealed her IF plan in May 2019 in an interview with a popular media platform. She is also a fan of the 16/8 variant of IF, where she fasts for 16 hours and feasts for the remaining 8 hours of the day. Talking about the benefits of this plan, she revealed that it makes her feel "more energized and "stronger" during her workout sessions.

The Lesley Leach Program

The warrior plan is the most extreme form of IF, and if you are following it in its truest form that involves a four-hour eating window, you need to plan your meal in a way that meets all of your nutrient requirements. However, if you are following a modified version of the warrior plan, you can add low-calorie drinks and snacks for your 20-hour-long fasting window. Two to three different items can be consumed during the fasting window. Therefore, your eating plan should look like this:

Morning Drink

Water with 1 tbsp ACV or lime juice

Low-calorie lunch

1 bowl of raw fruits or vegetables
Or
1 cup of yogurt
Or
1 glass of vegetable juice

Snack

Seaweed chips
Kale chips

Dinner (4-hour eating window)

The warrior diet is an intense plan and therefore requires you to employ an easy approach. You don't need to follow this diet every day. One or two cheat days are allowed in a week.

My warrior plan	**Day 1**	**Day 2**	**Day 3**	**Day 4**	**Day 5**	**Day 6**	**Day 7**
9 a.m.	Drink	Drink	Drink	**Cheat Day**	Drink	Drink	Drink
10 a.m.							
11 a.m.							
Noon.							
1 p.m.	Low-calorie lunch	Low-calorie lunch	Low-calorie lunch		Low-calorie lunch	Low-calorie lunch	Low-calorie lunch
2 p.m.							
3 p.m.							
4 p.m.			Snack				
5 p.m.	Snack	Snack			Snack	Snack	Snack
6 p.m.							
7 p.m.			**Eating window begins**				
8 p.m.	**Eating window begins**	**Eating window begins**			**Eating window begins**	**Eating window begins**	**Eating window begins**
9 p.m.							
10 p.m.							
11 p.m.			**Fasting window begins**				
Midnight.	**Fasting window begins**	**Fasting window begins**			**Fasting window begins**	**Fasting window begins**	**Fasting window begins**
1 a.m.							
2 a.m.							
3 a.m.							
4 a.m.							
5 a.m.							
6 a.m.							
7 a.m.							
8 a.m.							

You can use the following weekly planner to plan your warrior diet.

My warrior plan	**Day 1**	**Day 2**	**Day 3**	**Day 4**	**Day 5**	**Day 6**	**Day 7**
9 a.m. 10 a.m. 11 a.m. Noon. 1 p.m. 2 p.m. 3 p.m. 4 p.m. 5 p.m. 6 p.m. 7 p.m. 8 p.m. 9 p.m. 10 p.m. 11 p.m. Midnight. 1 a.m. 2 a.m. 3 a.m. 4 a.m. 5 a.m. 6 a.m. 7 a.m. 8 a.m.							

9

BONUS CHAPTER: RECIPES

▷ *Garlic Mushroom Chicken Thighs*

This is one of the most affordable and yummy keto meals. This chicken thigh recipe is a chicken thigh dipped in a spicy garlic mushroom sauce mixed with butter and herbs. Serve it with cauliflower rice or other low-carbohydrate options like zucchini noodles and mashed cauliflower.

Ingredients:

- 1/4 teaspoon of cracked black pepper
- 8 ounces of sliced brown mushrooms
- 1/2 teaspoon each of dried thyme
- 1 1/2 pounds of boneless skinless chicken thighs
- 1 teaspoon of onion powder
- 2 tablespoons of olive oil

- 1/2 teaspoon of Salt
- 1 teaspoon of garlic powder
- 1 tablespoon of butter
- 1 tablespoon of freshly chopped parsley
- 4 cloves of minced garlic

Instructions:

- Dry with a paper towel, reduce excessive fat, or keep it for taste.
- Combine the herbs, onion powder, salt, garlic powder, and pepper before coating the chicken evenly with the combined seasoning.
- Heat a tablespoon of olive or avocado oil in a skillet or large pan over medium-high heat, and sear the chicken thighs in batches till it becomes brown on either side and not pink in the middle. Do this for 8-10 minutes on each side.
- Add the rest of the oil, if necessary, for a second batch, then transfer the thighs to a plate, set them aside, and keep them warm.
- In the same pan or skillet, melt the butter, add the mushrooms, and season with salt and pepper. After that, cook it until it becomes soft, for 3 minutes.
- Add the thyme, garlic, parsley, and rosemary, then sauté until it becomes fragrant, for 1 minute.
- Add the chicken to the pan, taste it, and season it with salt and pepper to match your taste.

- Garnish with fresh parsley, and serve immediately.

▷ *Bacon Spinach Feta Chicken*

This recipe is low in carbohydrates and easy to prepare with spinach, feta cream sauce, and bacon. It can also be served with cauliflower rice for a delicious low-carb meal.

Ingredients:

- 6 boneless, skinless chicken thighs
- 5 ounces of baby spinach
- 6 strips of chopped bacon
- 2 cloves of minced garlic
- 1 cup of heavy cream
- 1/2 cup of crumbled feta
- 1 tablespoon of butter
- 1/2 cup of grated Parmesan
- Salt and pepper

Instructions:

- In a large skillet, cook the chopped bacon over medium heat until it's lightly crisped before removing it to a plate lined with a paper towel. Then allow it to drain, and leave the bacon grease in the pan.
- After that, season the chicken with pepper and salt, and place them in a pan. Cook for 6 minutes on each

side until they are cooked thoroughly, at the internal temperature of 165; put it on a plate, add butter, then allow it to melt.
- Add fresh garlic and cook for 1 minute or until it starts to savor. Add the spinach and lightly fry until it begins to wither for 2-3 minutes.
- Add Parmesan and heavy cream, then stir and cook until it becomes thick for 3 minutes. After that, return the bacon to the sauce, combine it all, place the chicken back in the pan and toss/flip to coat.
- To serve it, sprinkle the pan with crumbled feta, then serve it over cauliflower rice or zucchini noodles.

▷ *Chicken Liver with Peas and Radish*

Chicken liver is a unique dish you can enjoy in many ways. Chicken livers are rich in iron, vitamin A, and B12. Chicken livers have an interesting flavor but can easily be mixed with other ingredients to make them more palatable if you find the taste too strong or bitter. This dish is ideal for those looking for new ideas and low-carb meals.

Ingredients:

- 50 grams of chicken liver
- 40 grams of green peas cooked and cooled
- 1 green onion thinly sliced
- 30 grams thinly sliced radish
- 1/2 teaspoon of olive oil

- 1 teaspoon of soy sauce
- Splash of red wine vinegar

Instructions:

- Heat the oil, and add lightly-brown radishes and green onion.
- After that, remove them from the heat, and add them to the bowl of peas.
- Cook the liver in the same pan for 2 minutes on each side.
- Allow it to cool, then slice.
- Add liver to the bowl of vegetables, and toss with soy sauce and red wine vinegar.

▷ *Egg Scramble with Sweet Potatoes*

This Egg Scramble with Sweet Potatoes is the perfect healthy, hearty breakfast. It's loaded with sweet potatoes, peppers, onions, parsley, and scrambled eggs. This single simple dish is packed with savory flavors and is the perfect start to the day!

Ingredients:

- 2 teaspoons of chopped rosemary
- 4 large egg whites
- 1 (8 ounces) sweet potato, diced
- 4 large eggs

- 2 tablespoons of chopped chive
- 1/2 cup of chopped onion
- Salt
- Pepper

Instructions:

- Preheat the oven to 425°F.
- Toss the rosemary, onion, sweet potato, and salt and pepper on a baking sheet.
- Then drizzle with cooking spray and roast until it becomes tender, for 20 minutes.
- Meanwhile, in a medium bowl, whisk the eggs, a pinch of salt, egg whites, and pepper together. Then spurt a skillet with cooking spray and scramble the eggs on medium heat for 5 minutes.
- After that, sprinkle it with chopped chives.

▷ *Chicken, Broccoli & Beetroot Salad with Avocado Pesto*

This superfood dinner contains ingredients to boost your body, like red onion, nigella seeds, walnuts, avocado, and lemon oil.

Ingredients:

- 2 bunches of thin-stemmed broccoli
- 2 tsp avocado oil
- 3 skinless chicken breasts

- 1 red onion, thinly sliced
- 1 bag watercress
- 2 raw beetroots (about 175g), peeled and julienned or grated
- 1 tsp nigella seeds

For the avocado pesto:

- small pack basil
- 1 avocado
- ½ garlic cloves, crushed
- 25g walnut halves, crumbled
- 1 tbsp avocado oil
- juice and zest 1 lemon

Instructions:

- Add the broccoli to a large boiling pot and cook for about 4 minutes. Drain, then cool with cold water. Heat a skillet on medium, cook the broccoli in 1/2 teaspoon of olive oil, and grill for 2-3 minutes, turning, until lightly charred. Let it cool down. Lightly cover the chicken with the remaining oil and season. Add the chicken to the stove/grill for 4-6 minutes on each side or until cooked. Let cool, then cut or chop into large pieces.
- Next, prepare the pesto. Take the basil leaves and reserve a handful for decorating the salad. Put the

rest in a bowl or a food processor. Cut the avocado in half, spoon it out and place it in a food processor with the remaining ingredients and a little seasoning. Blend until smooth, then transfer to a small serving plate. Pour lemon juice over the sliced onions and let them sit to marinate.

- Stack the cress in a large bowl. Combine the broccoli and onion, along with the lemon juice. Top with the beets, but don't mix; add the chicken. Spread the basil leaves, lemon zest, and nigella seeds, set aside, then serve with the avocado pesto.

▷ ***The Best No Bun Hamburger***

This recipe is paleo and a keto-friendly hamburger with low calories.

INGREDIENTS:

For the Burgers:

- 2 cups of minced mushrooms
- 2 teaspoons of paprika
- 6 slices of sharp Cheddar (any hard cheese of your liking. Give Gouda a try too)
- 1 pound of ground beef
- 2 teaspoons of garlic powder
- 2 teaspoons of onion powder
- Salt and pepper, to taste

Toppings;

- Butter lettuce, red onions, sharp cheddar cheese, homemade mayonnaise, and avocado Arugula.

For dressed arugula;

- 3 cups of arugula
- 1/2 (half) of lemon juice.
- Salt and pepper

Instructions:

- Mix all the ingredients for the patty (meat, seasoning, and mushrooms) in a bowl, and form single patties, then place it on a grill or cook it in a skillet for 5-8 minutes per side until done or an internal temp of about 145. Top with your cheese of choice and other favs. Place the patty on your bed of arugula and all your toppings. Enjoy!

For arugula;

- Toss or flip the arugula with lemon juice, then rest for about 2 minutes. Serve.

▷ *Taco Stuffed Pepper Rings*

This recipe contains black beans, ground turkey, cheese and spices, etc.

Ingredients:

- 5 sweet bell peppers (cut them into 1-inch thick rings)
- 2 green chopped onions
- 1/2 pounds of cubed Monterey jack cheese
- 1/2 pounds of cubed cheddar cheese
- 2 tablespoons of Taco seasoning
- 1.5 pounds of ground turkey
- 1 egg
- 1/2 teaspoon of salt
- 1 can black beans

Instructions

- Preheat the oven to 400°c, then spray a baking sheet with cooking spray (I love duck fat spray) and put the pepper rings on top.
- Put all the ingredients in a bowl and mix. Then, divide the mixture between the pepper rings, cover with foil, and bake for about 30 minutes or until the meat is well cooked.
- Top the pepper rings with salsa, sour cream, and cilantro.

▷ *Turkey Taco Lettuce Wraps*

This turkey taco lettuce wrap is a recipe that is affordable, healthy, quick, and easy to prepare meal for dinner.

Ingredients:

- 1 teaspoon of ground cumin
- 2 cloves of garlic
- 1 tablespoon of olive oil
- 1/2 cup of low-sodium chicken broth
- 1 pound of lean ground turkey
- 1/2 teaspoon of paprika
- 1/2 cup of tomato sauce
- 3/4 cup of chopped yellow onion
- Salt and freshly ground black pepper
- 1 tablespoon of chili powder.
- A bunch of romaine

Instructions:

- Heat the olive oil in a non-stick skillet over medium-high heat, then add onion and saute for 2 minutes.
- After that, add turkey and garlic, season it with pepper salt, cook, toss/flip, and occasionally break up the turkey until it is thoroughly cooked, for about 5 minutes.
- Add chicken broth, chili powder, paprika, cumin, and tomato sauce, and allow it to boil for 5 minutes, then

cook for an additional 5 minutes until the sauce is reduced.
- Serve on top of romaine

▷ *Low-Carb Broccoli Cheese Soup*

This recipe is an inexpensive low carb dish that is tasty and satiating. It is also a great option for any autumn meal.

Ingredients:

- 3 cups of shredded cheddar cheese
- 2 tablespoons of butter (I prefer grass-fed)
- 1 teaspoon of garlic powder
- 1 stalk of chopped celery
- 3 pounds of broccoli florets (cut into bite-sized pieces)
- 3 cups of canned chicken stock or broth
- 1 teaspoon of paprika
- 1 yellow or white onion (chopped)
- Salt and pepper to taste
- 1 cup of heavy cream

Instructions:

- In a large pot, melt the butter over medium to high heat, then add the celery and onion until it softens.

- Add the broccoli, stir and cover it with stock, and allow it to boil until it becomes tender, for 10-15 minutes.
- To make the soup thick, set aside a cup of broccoli using a slotted spoon.
- Lower the heat, and stir in the garlic powder and paprika.
- After that, add the shredded cheddar cheese gradually, stir regularly, and continue to stir until it melts. Add in your cup of heavy cream.
- Use a blender or food processor, blend it until it becomes smooth, and stir in the broccoli you removed earlier.
- Serve, or add salt and pepper to taste.

▷ *Keto Salmon Cakes*

This recipe is healthy, nutritious, low-carb, and loaded with flavors.

Ingredients:

- 1/4 cup of sour cream
- 1 tablespoon of avocado oil
- 1/4 teaspoon of chili powder
- 5 pieces of pink salmon
- 1/4 teaspoon of garlic powder
- 1 egg
- 2 tablespoons of finely diced red onion
- Salt and pepper to taste

- 1 avocado
- 2 tablespoon avocado oil, to thin
- 1/2 of finely chopped jalapeno
- 1/2 of lemon juice
- 3 tablespoons of cilantro
- 1/4 cup of finely ground pork rinds
- 2 tablespoons of Sarayo or plain mayo
- Salt and pepper to taste

Instructions:

- Mix the jalapeno, egg, salmon, red onion, sarayo, and seasoning in a large bowl, then form patties with the mixture. It should produce 4 large or 5-6 small cakes. Lastly, press the patties into a plate of pork rinds to cover both sides.
- In a non-stick skillet, heat up the avocado oil, and cook the patties over medium heat for 4-5 minutes, or until each side becomes golden brown and crispy
- Top with lemon juice and a dollop of sour cream

▷ *Low-Carb Egg Salad*

This recipe is low in carbohydrates, delicious, and easy to prepare.

Ingredients:

- 1/4 teaspoon of sea salt

- 1 teaspoon of lemon juice
- 6 eggs
- 2 tablespoons of mayonnaise
- 1 teaspoon of Dijon mustard
- Kosher Salt
- Pepper
- Smoked Paprika

Instructions:

- Put the eggs in a medium saucepan gently, add cold water until the eggs are covered, at least 1 inch, then boil it for 10 minutes.
- After that, remove the eggs from the heat and let them cool; peel them under cold water.
- Add the eggs to a food processor to be chopped, then add mustard, mayonnaise, lemon juice, pepper, and salt, stir, taste, and adjust where necessary.
- I like to serve this atop lettuce leaves and sprinkle on some bacon bits and paprika or even a low-carb bun.

▷ *Keto Cheese Meatballs*

This recipe is easy to prepare, low-carb, tasty, and slightly cheesy.

Ingredients:

- 4 oz of Mozzarella or Cheddar cheese block

- 3 tablespoons of Parmesan cheese
- 1 pound of ground or minced beef
- 1 teaspoon of garlic powder
- 1/2 teaspoon of salt

Instructions:

- Slice the cheese into cubes. Mix the dry ingredients with ground beef. Now wrap the cubes of cheese with the meat mixture. However, 1cm x 1cm cheese cubes should produce approximately 9 balls.
- After that, put the cheese meatballs on a tray, oven-fry, air-fry, or pan-fry by covering it with a lid to spread the heat around evenly.
- Serve with a side salad

▷ ***Mexican Stuffed Peppers***

This recipe is typically combined by stuffing or filling the holes of the peppers and cooking them. This dish is a low-carb easy-to-prepare cuisine.

Ingredients:

- 2 cups of cheddar cheese
- 2 teaspoons of chili powder
- 3 cloves of minced garlic
- 2 cups of cooked Cauliflower Rice
- 4 red, yellow or green peppers

- 1 small diced yellow onion
- 1 can of diced tomatoes with peppers
- 1 teaspoon of cumin
- 1 pound of lean ground beef
- 1 can of enchilada sauce

Instructions:

- Preheat oven to 375°F. Wash and seed the bell peppers before cutting them into half from top to bottom. After that, please place them in a greased 9x13 inches baking dish,and set aside.
- Add ground beef, onion, and garlic to a pan over medium heat and cook and drain.
- Add your diced tomatoes, 2/3 cup of the enchilada sauce, chili powder, cumin, and stir.
- Then allow it to simmer for about 2-3 minutes. After that, please remove it from the heat and stir in the cooked or cauliflower rice.
- Divide the beef mixture into the pepper halves, then top it with the remaining cheese and enchilada sauce. After that, bake without covering it for about 30-35 minutes or until the peppers are cooked and the cheese melts.
- Top it with desired taco toppings and serve.

▷ *Carrot Zucchini Egg Cups*

Cook a batch of mini quiches quickly, and it will be satisfying to end an intermittent fasting period with the best meal.

Ingredients:

- 3/4 cup of packed grated zucchini
- 2 teaspoons coconut oil or any oil
- 4 large eggs, whisked
- 3/4 cup of packed grated carrots
- 1/4 cup of grated Monterrey Jack cheese*
- 1/4 teaspoon of SeaSalt
- 2 green shallots (onions), green ends trimmed off, white finely chopped (optional)

Instructions:

- Preheat the oven to 350°, and grease a mini cupcake pan.
- In a medium skillet, heat the oil over medium heat, add the zucchini, carrots, and shallots, and cook; stir for 7-9 minutes until the vegetables start to soften.
- After that, please remove it from the heat, and set it aside to cool down to room temperature.
- Mix all the vegetables, eggs, grated cheese, and salt in a large bowl.
- Spoon the mixture into a mini muffin pan.

- Bake for 15-18 minutes, and let the mini quiches cool off in the pan.
- After that, carefully remove it with a small knife or spatula.
- I like to top mine with hot sauce or salsa

▷ *Avocado Ricotta Power Toast*

This recipe is a quick and tasty lunch or snack that can be made gluten-free.

Ingredients:

- 1/4 ripe avocado, smashed
- 2 tablespoons of ricotta cheese
- 1 slice of whole-grain bread
- Pinch of crushed red pepper flakes
- Pinch of flaky sea salt.
- Pepper

Instructions:

- Toast the bread, and top it with avocado, ricotta, crushed red pepper flakes, pepper and sea salt.
- Then eat it with scrambled or hard-boiled eggs and a serving of fruit or yogurt.

YOUR CHANCE TO MAKE A DIFFERENCE

Now that you're fully equipped to use the power of intermittent fasting to reclaim your health and gain control over your weight, you're in the perfect position to help other women like you.

Simply by leaving your honest opinion of this book on Amazon, you'll show new readers where they can find a solution that will really work – without knocking their self-confidence along the way.

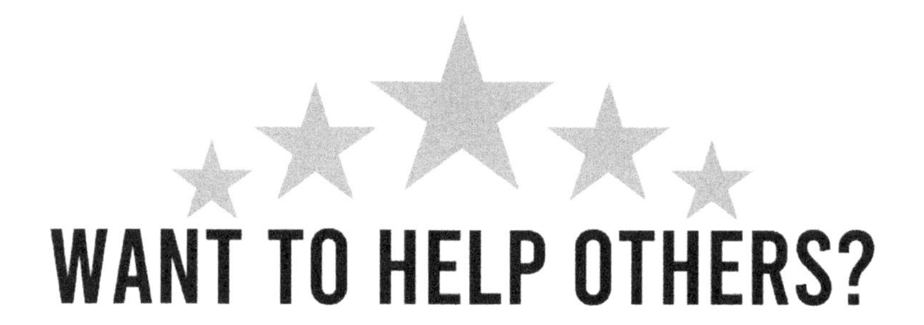

I can't thank you enough for your support. We all deserve to feel good about ourselves – and with the right information behind us, we will.

Scan the QR code below for a quick review!

CONCLUSION

Intermittent fasting is a lifesaver for all those women struggling to rein in their hormones and to slow down the detrimental changes that their bodies go through during the 50s. IF effectively deals with menopausal changes naturally without the involvement of strict diets, hormone replacement therapies, and intense workout regimens. In fact, IF combines the effects of all three of these schemes into a single package. It not only balances the hormone levels but assists in weight loss, maintains muscle mass, and lowers the risk of age-related illnesses simply by modulating your meal timings.

The fact that makes IF the best plan out there is its flexibility. It entails no strict rules. There are a number of IF methods ranging from the 14:1o plan to the intense warrior plan and extended fasting. Everyone can easily figure out an IF method that best fits their routine.

Women in their 50s stand to gain the most from IF. If you are someone going through menopausal changes, you must be facing several challenges in the form of excessive weight gain, muscle loss, brain fog, lethargy, and mood swings. IF can help you deal with all of these issues. Women suffering from hormone disorders and PCOS can also benefit from IF. An abundance of research has proven the efficacy of IF in lowering the risk of type 2 diabetes, CVD, and several types of cancer. In short, IF is a remedy that can effectively deal with all of your health concerns. Supplementing an IF routine with some healthy lifestyle changes like healthy eating and exercising can help your body to adjust easily to the IF routine and maximize its benefits.

Now that you are fully equipped with the basics of IF, you are all set to embark on a journey to regain your health, strength, and vigor. Remember, age is just a number, and you cannot let it claim some of the best years of your life. Sure, menopause and related changes will affect the quality of your life, but IF will help you recover from that at a fast pace. You are allowed to make mistakes on your way to becoming a pro at IF, and you *will* make mistakes. You might even consider quitting at the start, but you will soon start noticing a betterment in your health and energy levels, and you will never stop. I remember my initial days when I doubted the efficacy of IF and considered quitting every now and then. I committed several mistakes too, but I hope you won't go through the same–this fasting guide will make sure that doesn't happen. I wish you nothing but health and happiness.

Start your intermittent fasting journey today and reclaim your health. Happy fasting!

Just For You

A FREE GIFT TO MY READERS.
TOP 12 FAT LOSS FOODS WITH RECIPES!!

Just Scan the QR Code and download the PDF.

REFERENCES

Abbasi, B., Samadi, A., & Bazgir, B. (2020). The combined effect of high-intensity interval training and intermittent fasting on lipid profile and peroxidation in Wistar rats under high-fat diet. Sport Sciences for Health, 16(4), 645–652. https://doi.org/10.1007/s11332-020-00637-3

Abelsson, A. (2022, June 21). Intermittent fasting and strength training: The ultimate guide. StrengthLog. https://www.strengthlog.com/intermittent-fasting-and-strength-training/

Akram, M. (n.d.). HIIT and intermittent fasting: Pros, cons & workout - TheFitnessPhantom. Fitness Phantom. https://thefitnessphantom.com/hiit-and-intermittent-fasting

Anton, S. D., Moehl, K., Donahoo, W. T., Marosi, K., Lee, S. A., Mainous, A. G., Leeuwenburgh, C., & Mattson, M. P. (2018). Flipping the metabolic switch: Understanding and applying the health benefits of fasting. Obesity (Silver Spring, Md.), 26(2), 254–268. https://doi.org/10.1002/oby.22065

Arnarson, A. (2019, July 29). Antioxidants are explained in simple terms. Healthline. https://www.healthline.com/nutrition/antioxidants-explained#antioxidant-types

Arnason, T. G., Bowen, M. W., & Mansell, K. D. (2017). Effects of intermittent fasting on health markers in those with type 2 diabetes: A pilot study. World Journal of Diabetes, 8(4), 154. https://doi.org/10.4239/wjd.v8.i4.154

Bachman, J. L., Deitrick, R. W., & Hillman, A. R. (2016). Exercising in the fasted state reduced 24-hour energy intake in active male adults. Journal of Nutrition and Metabolism, 2016, 1–7. https://doi.org/10.1155/2016/1984198

Baier, L. (2020). 9 biggest intermittent fasting mistakes beginners make (and how to avoid them!). Www.youtube.com. https://www.youtube.com/watch?v=YAN6rlJVpGI

Bailey, E. (2021, November 30). The 5:2 intermittent fasting diet and weight loss. Healthline. https://www.healthline.com/health-news/how-the-52-intermittent-fasting-diet-can-help-you-lose-weight

Barnosky, A. R., Hoddy, K. K., Unterman, T. G., & Varady, K. A. (2014). Intermittent fasting vs daily calorie restriction for type 2 diabetes prevention: A review of human findings. Translational Research, 164(4), 302–311. https://doi.org/10.1016/j.trsl.2014.05.013

Berg, E. (2020). What really happens when we fast? Www.youtube.com. https://www.youtube.com/watch?v=vhmtoAYVRSo

Berry, K. D. (2020, March 10). 7 secrets to stop hunger pangs while fasting. Www.youtube.com. https://www.youtube.com/watch?v=aDESO3XqQ6E

Better Health Channel. (2012). Resistance training – health benefits. Vic.gov.au. https://www.betterhealth.vic.gov.au/health/healthyliving/resistance-training-health-benefits

Biddulph, M. (2022, June 2). Intermittent fasting 16:8: How-to, benefits and tips. Livescience.com. https://www.livescience.com/intermittent-fasting-16-8

Bjarnadottir, A. (2018). The beginner's guide to the 5:2 diet. Healthline. https://www.healthline.com/nutrition/the-5-2-diet-guide

Booth, L. (2022). Lifting weights while fasting: Should you do it? – fitbod. Fitbod. https://fitbod.me/blog/lifting-weights-while-fasting/

Boyers, L. (2020, July 20). Achieve your healthy weight by syncing meals with your internal clock. Mindbodygreen. https://www.mindbodygreen.com/articles/what-is-circadian-rhythm-fasting

Brick, S. (2021, May 21). Is alternate-day fasting really that good for you? We dig. Greatist. https://greatist.com/health/alternate-day-fasting

Brookie, K. L., Best, G. I., & Conner, T. S. (2018). Intake of raw fruits and vegetables is associated with better mental health than intake of processed fruits and vegetables. Frontiers in Psychology, 9. https://doi.org/10.3389/fpsyg.2018.00487

Buckingham, C., & 2020. (2020, September 14). 11 people who should never try intermittent fasting. Eat This Not That. https://www.eatthis.com/is-intermittent-fasting-safe/

Can a low-carb diet help you lose weight? (2020, November 18). Mayo Clinic. https://www.mayoclinic.org/healthy-lifestyle/weight-loss/in-depth/low-carb-diet/art-20045831

Cancer treatment centers of America. (2021, June 9). What you need to know about fasting and cancer. Cancer Treatment Centers of America. https://www.cancercenter.com/community/blog/2021/06/fasting-cancer

Castaneda, R. (2022, October 19). Intermittent fasting: Foods to eat and to limit. U.S. News. https://health.usnews.com/wellness/food/articles/intermittent-fasting-foods-to-eat-and-avoid

Center for Discovery. (2019, February 5). The dangers of intermittent fasting. Center for Discovery. https://centerfordiscovery.com/blog/the-dangers-of-intermittent-fasting/

Chander, R. (2018, September 14). I Tried Extreme Fasting by Eating Once a Day — Here's What Happen. Healthline. https://www.healthline.com/health/food-nutrition/one-meal-a-day-diet

Charkalis, D. M. (2017, November 24). Is this extreme form of intermittent fasting safe? Prevention. https://www.prevention.com/weight-loss/a20507557/extended-fasting/

Chiofalo, B., Laganà, A. S., Palmara, V., Granese, R., Corrado, G., Mancini, E., Vitale, S. G., Ban Frangež, H., Vrtačnik-Bokal, E., & Triolo, O. (2017). Fasting as possible complementary approach for polycystic ovary syndrome: Hope or hype? Medical Hypotheses, 105, 1–3. https://doi.org/10.1016/j.mehy.2017.06.013

Cienfuegos, S., Gabel, K., Kalam, F., Ezpeleta, M., Lin, S., & Varady, K. A. (2021). Changes in body weight and metabolic risk during time restricted feeding in premenopausal versus postmenopausal women. Experimental Gerontology, 154, 111545. https://doi.org/10.1016/j.exger.2021.111545

Cole, W. (2018, May 31). Intermittent fasting is confusing: Here's exactly when to eat. Mindbodygreen. https://www.mindbodygreen.com/articles/intermittent-fasting-diet-plan-how-to-schedule-meals

Conway, S.-M. (2020, April 3). Hungry during intermittent fasting? Learn how to deal with it. Simple.life Blog. https://simple.life/blog/intermittent-fast-without-being-hungry/

Coyle, D. (2018, July 22). Intermittent fasting for women: A beginner's guide. Healthline. https://www.healthline.com/nutrition/intermittent-fasting-for-women#best-types-for-women

Damas, F., Phillips, S., Vechin, F. C., & Ugrinowitsch, C. (2015). A review of resistance training-induced changes in skeletal muscle protein synthesis and their contribution to hypertrophy. Sports Medicine, 45(6), 801–807. https://doi.org/10.1007/s40279-015-0320-0

DeLauer, T. (2019, September 28). How to break a fast for women [female fasting instructions]. Www.youtube.com. https://www.youtube.com/watch?v=ZCaY8FYm2lk

Detriments of intermittent fasting. (2020, October 18). Newsweek. https://www.newsweek.com/amplify/vegin-out-why-you-shouldnt-try-intermittent-fasting

De Vantier, J. (2020a, January 20). The five common mistakes people make when intermittent fasting. Www.taste.com.au. https://www.taste.com.au/healthy/articles/five-common-mistakes-people-make-intermittent-fasting/gb5avhkn

De Vantier, J. (2020b, January 20). The five common mistakes people make when intermittent fasting. Www.taste.com.au. https://www.taste.com.au/healthy/articles/five-common-mistakes-people-make-intermittent-fasting/gb5avhkn

Diet review: Intermittent fasting for weight loss. (2018, January 16). The Nutrition Source. https://www.hsph.harvard.edu/nutritionsource/healthy-weight/diet-reviews/intermittent-fasting/

Eckelkamp, S. (2020, January 21). Intermittent fasting? Here's the right way to break your fast. Mindbodygreen. https://www.mindbodygreen.com/articles/intermittent-fasting-heres-right-way-to-break-your-fast

Ederer, J. (2020, August 2). What to drink and eat while intermittent fasting | PIQUE. Pique Blog. https://blog.piquelife.com/what-to-drink-while-intermittent-fasting/

Ekberg, S. (2022). What happens if you don't eat for 3 days? Www.youtube.com. https://www.youtube.com/watch?v=WOxgJE6QR2o&t=583s

Ellis, S. (2017, March 10). How should you exercise while you're intermittent fasting? Doctors weigh in. Mindbodygreen. https://www.mindbodygreen.com/articles/how-to-exercise-while-intermittent-fasting

Falcone, P. H., Tai, C.-Y., Carson, L. R., Joy, J. M., Mosman, M. M., McCann, T. R., Crona, K. P., Kim, M. P., & Moon, J. R. (2015). Caloric expenditure of aerobic, resistance, or combined high-intensity interval training using a hydraulic resistance system in healthy men. Journal of Strength and Conditioning Research, 29(3), 779–785. https://doi.org/10.1519/jsc.0000000000000661

Fasting. (2019). In Encyclopædia Britannica. https://www.britannica.com/topic/fasting

FitPro Team. (2020, October 23). Intermittent fasting men vs. women. FitPro Blog. https://www.fitpro.com/blog/intermittent-fasting-men-vs-women/

Fletcher, J. (2019, April 5). Intermittent fasting for weight loss: 5 tips to start. Www.medicalnewstoday.com. https://www.medicalnewstoday.com/articles/324882

Fletcher, S. W., & Colditz, G. A. (2002). Failure of estrogen plus progestin therapy for prevention. JAMA, 288(3), 366. https://doi.org/10.1001/jama.288.3.366

Folin, O., & Denis, W. (1915). On starvation and Obesity, with special reference to acidosis. Journal of Biological Chemistry, 21(1), 183–192. https://doi.org/10.1016/S0021-9258(18)88204-7

Garofalo, E. (n.d.). The beginner's guide to the warrior diet plan 2022. Healthcanal.com. Retrieved October 30, 2022, from https://www.healthcanal.com/life-style-fitness/warrior-diet-weight-loss-results

Geurin, L. (2021, December 23). 42 intermittent fasting quotes to motivate you. LoriGeurin.com | Wellness for Life. https://lorigeurin.com/intermittent-fasting-quotes/

Greenberg, J. A., & Geliebter, A. (2012). Coffee, hunger, and peptide YY. Journal of the American College of Nutrition, 31(3), 160–166. https://doi.org/10.1080/07315724.2012.10720023

Griffith, T. (2017, October 16). Fasting and cancer: The science behind this treatment method. Healthline. https://www.healthline.com/health/fasting-and-cancer#how-it-works

Gudden, J., Arias Vasquez, A., & Bloemendaal, M. (2021). The effects of intermittent fasting on brain and cognitive function. Nutrients, 13(9), 3166. https://doi.org/10.3390/nu13093166

Gunnars, K. (2020, April 20). Intermittent fasting 101 — The ultimate beginner's guide. Healthline. https://www.healthline.com/nutrition/intermittent-fasting-guide

Hajek, P., Przulj, D., Pesola, F., McRobbie, H., Peerbux, S., Phillips-Waller, A., Bisal, N., & Myers Smith, K. (2021). A randomised controlled trial of the 5:2 diet. PloS One, 16(11), e0258853. https://doi.org/10.1371/journal.pone.0258853

Hammond, N. (2020). The healthy mama weight loss program. Nicky Hammond Coaching. https://nickyhammond.com/wp-content/uploads/2020/02/Intermittent-Fasting-Worksheet.pdf

Hanka, S. (2021, July 2). 10 intermittent fasting benefits and potential risks. Www.trifectanutrition.com. https://www.trifectanutrition.com/blog/intermittent-fasting-benefits-and-potential-risks

Harris, S. (2020, January 5). What happens if you don't eat for a day? Timeline and effects. Www.medicalnewstoday.com. https://www.medicalnewstoday.com/articles/322065

Harvie, M., & Howell, A. (2017). Potential benefits and harms of intermittent energy restriction and intermittent fasting amongst obese, overweight and normal weight subjects—a narrative review of human and animal evidence. Behavioral Sciences, 7(4), 4. https://doi.org/10.3390/bs7010004

Harvie, M. N., Pegington, M., Mattson, M. P., Frystyk, J., Dillon, B., Evans, G., Cuzick, J., Jebb, S. A., Martin, B., Cutler, R. G., Son, T. G., Maudsley, S., Carlson, O. D., Egan, J. M., Flyvbjerg, A., & Howell, A. (2010). The effects of intermittent or continuous energy restriction on weight loss and metabolic disease risk markers: A randomized trial in young overweight women. International Journal of Obesity, 35(5), 714–727. https://doi.org/10.1038/ijo.2010.171

Heffernan, C. (2020, April 21). Guest Post: The History of Intermittent Fasting. Physical Culture Study. https://physicalculturestudy.com/2020/04/21/guest-post-the-history-of-intermittent-fasting/

Hoare, K. (2020, December 13). Intermittent fasting and PCOS: What a nutritionist wants you to know. Www.nutritionist-Resource.org.uk. https://www.nutritionist-resource.org.uk/blog/2020/12/13/intermittent-fasting-and-pcos-what-a-nutritionist-wants-you-to-know

How intermittent fasting can help with PCOS. (2021, February 3). Fertility Family. https://www.fertilityfamily.co.uk/blog/how-intermittent-fasting-can-help-with-pcos/

Intermittent fasting and ketogenic diet. (2018). ABC Keto. https://abcketo.com/intermittent-fasting/

Intermittent Fasting, Definition, Origins, Demographics, Description. (n.d.). Reference.jrank.org. https://reference.jrank.org/diets/Intermittent_Fasting.html

Intermittent fasting: How to curb your hunger. (2019, March 13). Lean Squad. https://lean-squad.com/blog/curb-hunger-if/

Intermittent fasting worksheet eating window fasting and awake fasting and asleep 12:12 fasting day. (2020). Metagenics Institute. https://www.

amipro.co.za/uploads/1/1/9/5/119531810/met3096-intermittent-fast ing-patient-handout.pdf

Is eating one meal a day safe? (2021, April 8). WebMD. https://www.webmd. com/diet/is-eating-one-meal-a-day-safe

Is intermittent fasting a safe diet for PCOS. (n.d.). Sydney's Leading Dietitians | Sports Dieticians | Nutritionists Providing Best Nutrition, Diet and Lifestyle Advices. https://www.thelifestyledietitian.com.au/blog/2020/9/7/pcos-and-intermittent-fasting

ISSA. (2022). Intermittent fasting: Women vs. men | ISSA. Www.issaonline.com. https://www.issaonline.com/blog/post/this-hot-diet-trend-is-not-recommended-for-women

Jennifer Aniston and Reese Witherspoon reveal fasting is the secret behind their youthful looks. (2022). The Hits. https://www.thehits.co.nz/spy/jennifer-aniston-and-reese-witherspoon-reveal-fasting-is-the-secret-behind-their-youthful-looks/

John Hopkins Medicine. (2021). Intermittent Fasting: What is it, and how does it work? Www.hopkinsmedicine.org. https://www.hopkinsmedicine.org/health/wellness-and-prevention/intermittent-fasting-what-is-it-and-how-does-it-work

Johnson, J. (2019, January 28). The 5:2 diet: A guide and meal plan. Www.medicalnewstoday.com. https://www.medicalnewstoday.com/arti cles/324303

Johnstone, A., Faber, P., Gibney, E., Elia, M., Horgan, G., Golden, B., & Stubbs, R. (2002). Effect of an acute fast on energy compensation and feeding behaviour in lean men and women. International Journal of Obesity, 26(12), 1623–1628. https://doi.org/10.1038/sj.ijo.0802151

Just skip a meal. (2022). Metabolic Research Center. https://www.emetabolic.com/locations/centers/cary/blog/weight-loss/spontaneous-meal-skip ping-is-an-informal-fasting-protocol/

Kalam, F., Gabel, K., Cienfuegos, S., Ezpeleta, M., Wiseman, E., & Varady, K. A. (2021). Alternate day fasting combined with a low carbohydrate diet: Effect on sleep quality, duration, insomnia severity and risk of obstructive sleep apnea in adults with obesity. Nutrients, 13(1), 211. https://doi.org/10.3390/nu13010211

Kerndt, P. R., Naughton, J. L., Driscoll, C. E., & Loxterkamp, D. A. (1982). Fasting: The history, pathophysiology and complications. The Western

Journal of Medicine, 137(5), 379–399. https://pubmed.ncbi.nlm.nih.gov/6758355/

Kubala, J. (2021, April 23). 9 potential intermittent fasting side effects. Healthline. https://www.healthline.com/nutrition/intermittent-fasting-side-effects#8.-Dehydration

Lawler, M. (2022, February 10). 12 burning questions about intermittent fasting, answered | everyday health. EverydayHealth.com. https://www.everydayhealth.com/diet-nutrition/burning-questions-about-intermittent-fasting-answered/

Leech, J. (2017, December 11). 5 stats that show why intermittent fasting is powerful for weight loss | diet vs disease. Diet vs Disease. https://www.dietvsdisease.org/intermittent-fasting-is-powerful-for-weight-loss/

Leffler, S. (2020, May 7). Intermittent fasting tips from Kourtney Kardashian: Drink green tea, more. Us Weekly. https://www.usmagazine.com/food/pictures/intermittent-fasting-tips-from-kourtney-kardashian-pics/stick-to-satiating-meals/

Leonard, J. (2020, January 17). 16:8 intermittent fasting: Benefits, how-to, and tips. Www.medicalnewstoday.com. https://www.medicalnewstoday.com/articles/327398

Lett, R. (2021, September 8). Guide to managing hunger, while intermittent fasting. Www.span.health. https://www.span.health/blog/guide-to-hunger-while-intermittent-fasting

Lindberg, S. (2018a, September 11). Can you lose weight faster by exercising on an empty stomach? Healthline. https://www.healthline.com/health/fitness-exercise/fasted-cardio-when-to-eat-workout#2.-Skip-it:-Eating-before-a-cardio-workout-is-essential-if-youre-trying-to-add-muscle-mass

Lindberg, S. (2018b, October 26). How to exercise safely during intermittent fasting. Healthline. https://www.healthline.com/health/how-to-exercise-safely-intermittent-fasting#exercising-and-fasting-safely

Lin, S., Oliveira, M. L., Gabel, K., Kalam, F., Cienfuegos, S., Ezpeleta, M., Bhutani, S., & Varady, K. A. (2020). Does the weight loss efficacy of alternate day fasting differ according to sex and menopausal status? Nutrition, Metabolism and Cardiovascular Diseases, 31(2). https://doi.org/10.1016/j.numecd.2020.10.018

Longo, V. D., & Panda, S. (2016). Fasting, circadian rhythms, and time-restricted feeding in healthy lifespan. Cell Metabolism, 23(6), 1048–1059. https://doi.org/10.1016/j.cmet.2016.06.001

Mann, D. (2021, March 25). 50 health secrets every woman over 50 should know. The Healthy. https://www.thehealthy.com/aging/healthy-aging/health-secrets-women-over-50/

Matthews, M., & Pandika, M. (2019, January 27). What are the risks and side effects of intermittent fasting? Men's Health; Men's Health. https://www.menshealth.com/health/a26052066/side-effects-of-intermittent-fasting/

Mattson, M. P., Moehl, K., Ghena, N., Schmaedick, M., & Cheng, A. (2018). Intermittent metabolic switching, neuroplasticity and brain health. Nature Reviews Neuroscience, 19(2), 80–80. https://doi.org/10.1038/nrn.2017.156

Mayo Clinic. (2019). Menopause weight gain: Stop the middle age spread. Mayo Clinic. https://www.mayoclinic.org/healthy-lifestyle/womens-health/in-depth/menopause-weight-gain/art-20046058

McCarthy, N. (2020, December 16). These were the leading causes of death worldwide in 2019. World Economic Forum. https://www.weforum.org/agenda/2020/12/cause-of-death-dying-disease-health

Meat, poultry, fish, dry beans, eggs, and nuts. (n.d.). Www.umass.edu. https://www.umass.edu/nibble/infofile/meats.html

Merriam-Webster. (n.d.). HIIT. In Merriam-Webster.com dictionary. Retrieved November 1, 2022, from https://www.merriam-webster.com/dictionary/HIIT

Merriam-Webster. (n.d.). Strength training. In Merriam-Webster.com dictionary. Retrieved November 2, 2022, from https://www.merriam-webster.com/dictionary/strength%20training

Midland, N. (2020, September 30). 18:6 intermittent fasting: Can eating only 2 full meals help you slim down? BetterMe Blog. https://betterme.world/articles/186-intermittent-fasting/

Migala, J. (2020, April 20). 7 types of intermittent fasting: Which is best for you? | everyday health. EverydayHealth.com. https://www.everydayhealth.com/diet-nutrition/diet/types-intermittent-fasting-which-best-you/

Migala, J. (2021, November 18). OMAD diet: Safety, health benefits, risks, and more. EverydayHealth.com. https://www.everydayhealth.com/diet-nutrition/omad-diet/

Miglio, C., Chiavaro, E., Visconti, A., Fogliano, V., & Pellegrini, N. (2008).

Effects of different cooking methods on nutritional and physicochemical characteristics of selected vegetables. Journal of Agricultural and Food Chemistry, 56(1), 139–147. https://doi.org/10.1021/jf072304b

Moon, S., Kang, J., Kim, S. H., Chung, H. S., Kim, Y. J., Yu, J. M., Cho, S. T., Oh, C.-M., & Kim, T. (2020). Beneficial effects of time-restricted eating on metabolic diseases: A systemic review and meta-analysis. Nutrients, 12(5), 1267. https://doi.org/10.3390/nu12051267

Morales-Brown, L. (2020, June 11). Intermittent fasting and exercise: How to do it safely. Www.medicalnewstoday.com. https://www.medicalnewstoday.com/articles/intermittent-fasting-and-working-out#planning

Mudge, L. (2022, May 19). Intermittent fasting for women: Is it safe? Livescience.com. https://www.livescience.com/intermittent-fasting-for-women

Nerd fitness intermittent fasting blueprint. (n.d.). Nerd Fitness. https://www.nerdfitness.com/wp-content/uploads/2017/07/Intermittent-Fasting.pdf

Nutrafol Team. (2019, October 11). Women need to know this before trying intermittent fasting. Nutrafol. https://nutrafol.com/blog/intermittent-fasting-men-women/

Nyuar, K. B., Khalil, A. K. H., & Crawford, M. A. (2012). Dietary intake of Sudanese women: A comparative assessment of nutrient intake of displaced and non-displaced women. Nutrition and Health, 21(2), 131–144. https://doi.org/10.1177/0260106012467244

Panoff, L. (2019, September 26). What breaks a fast? Foods, drinks, and supplements. Healthline. https://www.healthline.com/nutrition/what-breaks-a-fast

Parker, K. (2021, June 2). The effect of intermittent fasting on your brain. Aviv Clinics USA. https://aviv-clinics.com/blog/nutrition/the-effect-of-intermittent-fasting-on-your-brain/

Preiato, D. (2019, May 23). 48-Hour fast: How-To, benefits, and downsides. Healthline. https://www.healthline.com/nutrition/48-hour-fasting

Putka, S. (2021, July 9). Male and female bodies can respond differently to intermittent fasting. Inverse. https://www.inverse.com/mind-body/intermittent-fasting-difference-men-women

Rankin, J. (2022, October 17). Alternate-day fasting: A beginner's guide. Diet Doctor. https://www.dietdoctor.com/weight-loss/alternate-day-fasting

Redman, L. M., & Ravussin, E. (2011). Caloric restriction in humans: Impact on physiological, psychological, and behavioral outcomes. Antioxidants & Redox Signaling, 14(2), 275–287. https://doi.org/10.1089/ars.2010.3253

Remes, O., Brayne, C., van der Linde, R., & Lafortune, L. (2016). A systematic review of reviews on the prevalence of anxiety disorders in adult populations. Brain and Behavior, 6(7). https://doi.org/10.1002/brb3.497

Revelant, J. (n.d.). Is intermittent fasting safe for people with diabetes? | everyday health. EverydayHealth.com. https://www.everydayhealth.com/type-2-diabetes/diet/intermittent-fasting-safe-people-with-diabetes/

Rizzo, N. (2018, May 7). What foods are best to eat on an intermittent fasting diet? Greatist; Greatist. https://greatist.com/eat/what-to-eat-on-an-inter mittent-fasting-diet

Rohner, M., Heiz, R., Feldhaus, S., & Bornstein, S. R. (2021). Hepatic-Metabolite-Based intermittent fasting enables a sustained reduction in insulin resistance in type 2 diabetes and metabolic syndrome. Hormone and Metabolic Research, 53(08), 529–540. https://doi.org/10.1055/a-1510-8896

Ryan. (2021, March 25). Intermittent fasting meal plan. Ryan and Alex Duo Life. https://www.ryanandalex.com/intermittent-fasting-meal-plan/

Rymer, J., Wilson, R., & Ballard, K. (2003). Making decisions about hormone replacement therapy. BMJ : British Medical Journal, 326(7384), 322–326. https://www.ncbi.nlm.nih.gov/pmc/articles/PMC1125186/

Rynders, C. A., Thomas, E. A., Zaman, A., Pan, Z., Catenacci, V. A., & Melanson, E. L. (2019). Effectiveness of intermittent fasting and time-restricted feeding compared to continuous energy restriction for weight loss. Nutrients, 11(10), 2442. https://doi.org/10.3390/nu11102442

Sadhukhan, P. (2017, November 24). The warrior diet plan – A complete guide. STYLECRAZE. https://www.stylecraze.com/articles/warrior-diet-plan-a-complete-guide/

Scher, B. (2019, April 25). Your complete guide to intermittent fasting. Diet Doctor. https://www.dietdoctor.com/intermittent-fasting

Schoenfeld, B. J., Aragon, A. A., Wilborn, C. D., Krieger, J. W., & Sonmez, G. T. (2014). Body composition changes associated with fasted versus non-fasted aerobic exercise. Journal of the International Society of Sports Nutrition, 11(1). https://doi.org/10.1186/s12970-014-0054-7

Seimon, R. V., Roekenes, J. A., Zibellini, J., Zhu, B., Gibson, A. A., Hills, A. P., Wood, R. E., King, N. A., Byrne, N. M., & Sainsbury, A. (2015). Do intermittent diets provide physiological benefits over continuous diets for weight loss? A systematic review of clinical trials. Molecular and Cellular Endocrinology, 418, 153–172. https://doi.org/10.1016/j.mce.2015.09.014

Seitz, A. (2021, June 28). Why starving yourself isn't a good idea for weight loss. Healthline. https://www.healthline.com/nutrition/starving-yourself#How-to-Lose-Weight-Fast-in-3-Simple-Steps

Sethmini. (2021, July 6). Difference between fasting and starving. Compare the Difference between Similar Terms. https://www.differencebetween.com/difference-between-fasting-and-starving/

Sharma, A., Madaan, V., & Petty, F. D. (2006). Exercise for mental health. Primary Care Companion to the Journal of Clinical Psychiatry, 8(2), 106. https://doi.org/10.4088/pcc.v08n0208a

Shemek, L. (2021, April). Top 9 foods to eat while intermittent fasting according to A nutritionist. Pk.iherb.com. https://pk.iherb.com/blog/best-intermittent-fasting-foods/1238

Shillington, P. (2017, January 4). Never too late: Building muscle and strength after 60. Resource | Baptist Health South Florida. https://baptisthealth.net/baptist-health-news/never-late-building-muscle-strength-60/

Siefert, R. (2020, March 2). Ways you didn't know your body changes after 50. The Daily Meal. https://www.thedailymeal.com/healthy-eating/body-changes-after-50-gallery

Silver, N. (2017, December 15). What happens if you don't eat for a day? Healthline. https://www.healthline.com/health/food-nutrition/what-happens-if-you-dont-eat-for-a-day

Simone de beauvoir quote: "To lose confidence in one's body is to lose confidence in oneself.". (n.d.). Quotefancy: Wallpapers With Inspirational Quotes. https://quotefancy.com/quote/969595/Simone-de-Beauvoir-To-lose-confidence-in-one-s-body-is-to-lose-confidence-in-oneself

Skolnik, N. S., & King, M. (2005). Dietary guidelines for Americans 2005. Family Practice News, 35(14), 58. https://doi.org/10.1016/s0300-7073(05)71075-6

Stanton, B. (2021, January 10). Extended fasting: Benefits, tips, and how to get started. KETO-MOJO. https://keto-mojo.com/article/extended-fasting-benefits/

Stanton, B. (2022, February). Intermittent fasting for women over 50: 7 tips for success. Carb Manager. https://www.carbmanager.com/article/ygj3xheaaawus2xa/intermittent-fasting-for-women-over-50-7-tips-for/

Stewart, W. K., & Fleming, L. W. (1973). Features of a successful therapeutic fast of 382 days' duration. Postgraduate Medical Journal, 49(569), 203–209. https://doi.org/10.1136/pgmj.49.569.203

Stote, K. S., Baer, D. J., Spears, K., Paul, D. R., Harris, G. K., Rumpler, W. V., Strycula, P., Najjar, S. S., Ferrucci, L., Ingram, D. K., Longo, D. L., & Mattson, M. P. (2007). A controlled trial of reduced meal frequency without caloric restriction in healthy, normal-weight, middle-aged adults. The American Journal of Clinical Nutrition, 85(4), 981–988. https://www.ncbi.nlm.nih.gov/pmc/articles/PMC2645638/

Streit, L., & Link, R. (2018, September 4). 16/8 intermittent fasting: A beginner's guide. Healthline; Healthline Media. https://www.healthline.com/nutrition/16-8-intermittent-fasting

Sundfør, T. M., Svendsen, M., & Tonstad, S. (2018). Effect of intermittent versus continuous energy restriction on weight loss, maintenance and cardiometabolic risk: A randomized 1-year trial. Nutrition, Metabolism and Cardiovascular Diseases, 28(7), 698–706. https://doi.org/10.1016/j.numecd.2018.03.009

The guide to 18:6 intermittent fasting. (2022, February 8). Mdrive. https://www.mdriveformen.com/blogs/the-driven/18-6-intermittent-fasting-schedule

Tinsley, G., & Read, T. (2021, December 20). HIIT benefits: 7 reasons to try high intensity interval training. Healthline. https://www.healthline.com/nutrition/benefits-of-hiit#how-to-get-started

Tobey, J. A. (1951). The biology of human starvation. American Journal of Public Health and the Nations Health, 41(2), 236–237. https://www.ncbi.nlm.nih.gov/pmc/articles/PMC1526048/

Torelli, P., & Manzoni, G. C. (2010). Fasting headache. Current Pain and Headache Reports, 14(4), 284–291. https://doi.org/10.1007/s11916-010-0119-5

Trumpfeller, G. (2020, May 15). 7 most common intermittent fasting mistakes. Simple.life Blog. https://simple.life/blog/intermittent-fasting-mistakes/

Varady, K. A., Bhutani, S., Klempel, M. C., Kroeger, C. M., Trepanowski, J. F.,

Haus, J. M., Hoddy, K. K., & Calvo, Y. (2013). Alternate day fasting for weight loss in normal weight and overweight subjects: A randomized controlled trial. Nutrition Journal, 12(1). https://doi.org/10.1186/1475-2891-12-146

Varady, K. A., Cienfuegos, S., Ezpeleta, M., & Gabel, K. (2021). Cardiometabolic benefits of intermittent fasting. Annual Review of Nutrition, 41(1), 333–361. https://doi.org/10.1146/annurev-nutr-052020-041327

Vera, K. (2018, December 17). Difference between fasting & starving. Healthy Eating | SF Gate. https://healthyeating.sfgate.com/difference-between-fasting-starving-11753.html

Vetter, C. (2022). Intermittent fasting: What can you eat or drink? Joinzoe.com. https://joinzoe.com/learn/what-to-eat-or-drink-while-intermittent-fasting

Vitamins and minerals. (2017). Nhsinform.scot. https://www.nhsinform.scot/healthy-living/food-and-nutrition/eating-well/vitamins-and-minerals

Vitti, A. (2018, October 23). Intermittent fasting and hormonal health: What you need to know. Flo Living. https://www.floliving.com/intermittent-fasting/

Waterhouse, J. (2020, October 16). 9 celebrities who swear by intermittent fasting. Marie Claire. https://www.marieclaire.com.au/intermittent-fasting-celebrities

Watkins, E., & Serpell, L. (2016). The psychological effects of short-term fasting in healthy women. Frontiers in Nutrition, 3. https://doi.org/10.3389/fnut.2016.00027

Weeks, C. (2019, February 13). 20 best foods to eat while intermittent fasting. Eat This Not That; Eat This Not That. https://www.eatthis.com/intermittent-fasting-diet-foods/

Weeratunga, P., Jayasinghe, S., Perera, Y., Jayasena, G., & Jayasinghe, S. (2014). Per capita sugar consumption and prevalence of diabetes mellitus – global and regional associations. BMC Public Health, 14(1). https://doi.org/10.1186/1471-2458-14-186

Werner, C. (2021, March 31). Intermittent fasting with diabetes: A guide. Healthline. https://www.healthline.com/health/type-2-diabetes/intermittent-fasting-and-diabetes-safe#is-it-safe

What to know about intermittent fasting for women after 50. (n.d.). WebMD.

https://www.webmd.com/healthy-aging/what-to-know-about-intermittent-fasting-for-women-after-50

Wilhelmi de Toledo, F., Grundler, F., Bergouignan, A., Drinda, S., & Michalsen, A. (2019). Safety, health improvement and well-being during a 4 to 21-day fasting period in an observational study including 1422 subjects. PLOS ONE, 14(1), e0209353. https://doi.org/10.1371/journal.pone.0209353

Wilhelmi de Toledo, F., Grundler, F., Sirtori, C. R., & Ruscica, M. (2020). Unraveling the health effects of fasting: a long road from obesity treatment to healthy life span increase and improved cognition. Annals of Medicine, 52(5), 147–161. https://doi.org/10.1080/07853890.2020.1770849

Wrona, T. (2022, January 3). Alternate day fasting: Schedule, benefits, and meal plan. Dr. Robert Kiltz. https://www.doctorkiltz.com/alternate-day-fasting/

Zeratsky, K. (2021, October 9). What to know before you juice. Mayo Clinic. https://www.mayoclinic.org/healthy-lifestyle/nutrition-and-healthy-eating/expert-answers/juicing/faq-20058020

Zhao, Y., Jia, M., Chen, W., & Liu, Z. (2022). The neuroprotective effects of intermittent fasting on brain aging and neurodegenerative diseases via regulating mitochondrial function. Free Radical Biology and Medicine, 182, 206–218. https://doi.org/10.1016/j.freeradbiomed.2022.02.021

Made in the USA
Las Vegas, NV
25 January 2023

66233586R00125